220|9800561S
14|11 99 ✱

362
.018
/Hea

D0317585

LEARNING AND INFORMATION
SERVICES
UNIVERSITY OF CUMBRIA

Health Services Research Methods

Health Services Research Methods: A guide to best practice

Edited by

Nick Black

Professor of Health Services Research, London School of Hygiene and Tropical Medicine, UK

John Brazier

Director, Sheffield Health Economics Group, School of Health and Related Research, University of Sheffield, UK

Ray Fitzpatrick

Professor of Public Health, University of Oxford, UK

Barnaby Reeves

Senior Lecturer in Epidemiology, London School of Hygiene and Tropical Medicine, UK

© BMJ Books 1998
BMJ Books is an imprint of the BMJ Publishing Group

All rights reserved. No part of this publication may be reproduced, stored in a retrieval system, or transmitted, in any form or by any means, electronic, mechanical, photocopying, recording and/or otherwise, without the prior written permission of the publishers.

First published in 1998
by BMJ Books, BMA House, Tavistock Square,
London WC1H 9JR

British Library Cataloguing in Publication Data

A catalogue record for this book is available from the
British Library

ISBN 0–7279–1275–5

UNIVERSITY OF
NORTHUMBRIA AT NEWCASTLE
LIBRARY

ITEM No.	CLASS No.
20 091 959 01	362.018 HEA

Typeset, printed, and bound in Great Britain by
Latimer Trend & Company Ltd, Plymouth

Contents

Appendices

Contributors

Keith Abrams *Senior Lecturer in Medical Statistics, Department of Epidemiology and Public Health, University of Leicester*

Deborah Ashby *Professor of Medical Statistics, Department of Environmental and Preventive Medicine, Queen Mary and Westfield College, University of London*

Richard E Ashcroft *Lecturer in Ethics in Medicine, Centre for Ethics in Medicine, University of Bristol*

Janet Askham *Professor of Social Gerontology, Institute of Gerontology, GKT School of Medicine, University of London*

Chris Bain *Reader in Social and Preventive Medicine, Department of Social and Preventive Medicine, University of Queensland, Australia*

Claire Bamford *Research Associate, Centre for Health Services Research, University of Newcastle*

Lucinda J Billingham *Research Fellow, Department of Epidemiology and Public Health, University of Leicester*

Andrew MS Black *Senior Lecturer in Anaesthetics, Department of Anaesthesia, University of Bristol*

Nick Black *Professor of Health Services Research, Health Services Research Unit, London School of Hygiene and Tropical Medicine, University of London*

John Bond *Professor of Health Services Research, Centre for Health Services Research, University of Newcastle*

D Jane Bower *Director, Kinnell Technologies, Edinburgh*

David A Braunholtz *Senior Research Fellow, Department of Public Health and Epidemiology, University of Birmingham*

John Brazier *Director, Sheffield Health Economics Group, School of Health and Related Research, University of Sheffield*

John A Brebner *Senior Lecturer, Department of General Practice and Primary Care, University of Aberdeen*

Andrew H Briggs *Research Training Fellow, Health Economics Research Centre, University of Oxford*

Annie Britton *Research Fellow, Health Services Research Unit, London School of Hygiene and Tropical Medicine, University of London*

Philip J Brown *Professor of Medical Statistics, Institute of Mathematics and Statistics, University of Kent at Canterbury*

CONTRIBUTORS

Peter GJ Burney *Professor of Public Health, Department of Public Health Medicine, GKT School of Medicine, University of London*

Martin J Buxton *Director, Health Economics Research Group, Brunel University*

John A Cairns *Director, Health Economics Research Unit, University of Aberdeen*

David W Chadwick *Professor of Neurology, Department of Neurological Sciences, University of Liverpool*

Susan Chinn *Reader in Medical Statistics, GKT School of Medicine, University of London*

Stephen RL Clark *Professor of Philosophy, Department of Philosophy, University of Liverpool*

Carl E Counsell *Clinical Research Fellow, Department of Clinical Neurosciences, University of Edinburgh*

Claire Davey *Research Assistant, Department of Community Medicine and General Practice, Monash University, Melbourne*

Mark Deverill *Research Associate, Sheffield Health Economics Group, School of Health and Related Research, University of Sheffield*

Robert Dingwall *Professor of Sociology, School of Sociology and Social Policy, University of Nottingham*

Allan Donner *Professor and Chairman, Department of Epidemiology and Biostatistics, University of Western Ontario, Canada*

Richard HT Edwards *Director, Wales Office of Research and Development in Health and Social Care, Cardiff*

Sarah JL Edwards *Research Fellow, Department of Public Health and Epidemiology, University of Birmingham*

Ray Fitzpatrick *Professor of Public Health and Primary Care, Institute of Health Sciences, University of Oxford*

Nick Freemantle *Senior Research Fellow, Medicines Evaluation Group, Centre for Health Economics, University of York*

Lucy J Frith *Lecturerer in Health Care Ethics, Department of Primary Care, University of Liverpool*

John Gabbay *Professor of Public Health, Wessex Institute for Health Research and Development, University of Southampton*

Andrew Garratt *Research Fellow, Department of Health Sciences and Clinical Evaluation, University of York*

William J Gillespie *Professor of Orthopaedic Surgery, Department of Orthopaedic Surgery, University of Edinburgh*

Adrian M Grant *Director, Health Services Research Unit, University of Aberdeen*

Alastair M Gray *Director, Health Economics Research Centre, University of Oxford*

Martin C Gulliford *Senior Lecturer in Public Health, Department of Public Health Medicine, GKT School of Medicine, University of London*

Emma Harvey *Research Fellow, Department of Health Sciences and Clinical Evaluation, University of York*

Ian M Harvey *Professor of Health Services Research, University of East Anglia*

Jenny Hewison *Senior Lecturer, Department of Psychology, University of Leeds*

Jane L Hutton *Senior Lecturer in Statistics, Department of Statistics, University of Newcastle*

Jennifer C Jackson *Director, Centre for Business and Professional Ethics, University of Leeds*

Ann Jacoby *Principal Research Associate, Centre for Health Services Research, University of Newcastle*

Katharine Johnston *Research Fellow, Health Economics Research Group, Brunel University*

David R Jones *Professor of Medical Statistics, Department of Epidemiology and Public Health, University of Leicester*

Sandra Kiauka *Research Fellow, Medical Statistics Unit, University of Edinburgh*

Donna Lamping *Senior Lecturer in Psychology, Health Services Research Unit, London School of Hygiene and Tropical Medicine, University of London*

Richard Lilford *Professor of Health Services Research, Department of Public Health and Epidemiology, University of Birmingham*

Elaine McColl *Senior Research Associate, Centre for Health Services Research, University of Newcastle*

Lorna McKee *Director of Research, Department of Management Studies, University of Aberdeen*

Martin McKee *Professor of European Public Health, Health Services Research Unit, London School of Hygiene and Tropical Medicine, University of London*

Rachel R MacLehose *Environmental Epidemiologist, Medical Toxicology Unit, Guy's and St Thomas' Hospital Trust, London*

Klim McPherson *Professor of Public Health Epidemiology, Cancer and Public Health Unit, London School of Hygiene and Tropical Medicine, University of London*

Theresa Marteau *Professor of Health Psychology, Psychology and Genetics Research Group, GKT School of Medicine, University of London*

James Mason, *Research Fellow, Medicines Evaluation Group, Centre for Health Economics, University of York*

Ruairidh Milne *Director, NHS NCCHTA, University of Southampton*

Graham Mowatt *Review Group Co-ordinator, Health Services Research Unit, University of Aberdeen*

Elizabeth Murphy *Senior Lecturer, School of Sociology and Social Policy, University of Nottingham*

Maggie Murphy *Research Fellow, Health Services Research Unit, London School of Hygiene and Tropical Medicine, University of London*

Jonathan P Myles *Research Fellow, MRC Biostatistics Unit, Institute of Public Health, University of Cambridge*

Robin J Prescott *Director, Medical Statistics Unit, University of Edinburgh*

Barnaby C Reeves *Senior Lecturer in Epidemiology, Health Services Research Unit, London School of Hygiene and Tropical Medicine, University of London*

Glenn Robert *Research Associate, Wessex Institute for Health Research and Development, University of Southampton*

Susan Ross, *Senior Research Fellow, Health Services Research Unit, University of Aberdeen*

Ian T Russell *Professor, Department of Health Sciences and Clinical Evaluation, University of York*

Colin Sanderson *Senior Lecturer in Health Services Research, Health Services Research Unit, London School of Hygiene and Tropical Medicine, University of London*

Trevor A Sheldon *Professor, York Health Policy Group, University of York*

Fujian Song *Senior Research Fellow, NHS Centre for Reviews and Dissemination, University of York*

Jennifer Soutter *Research Associate, Centre for Health Services Research, University of Newcastle*

David J Spiegelhalter *Senior Statistician, MRC Biostatistics Unit, Institute of Public Health, University of Cambridge*

Jonathan AC Sterne, *Senior Lecturer in Medical Statistics, GKT School of Medicine, University of London*

Andrew Stevens *Professor of Public Health, Department of Public Health and Epidemiology, University of Birmingham*

Alexander J Sutton *Research Associate, Department of Epidemiology and Public Health, University of Leicester*

Lois Thomas *Research Associate, Centre for Health Services Research, University of Newcastle*

Roger Thomas *Research Director, Social and Community Planning Research, London*

Mary Ann Thomson *Assistant Clinical Professor, School of Rehabilitation Science, McMaster University, Ontario, Canada*

Jim Thornton *Senior Lecturer, Institute of Epidemiology, University of Leeds*

Obioha C Ukoumunne *Research Associate in Medical Statistics, GKT School of Medicine, University of London*

Sarah J White *Research Assistant, Department of Mathematics, University of Liverpool*

Frederick M Wolf *Professor, Department of Health Services, School of Public Health and Community Medicine, University of Washington School of Medicine, Seattle, Washington, USA*

John Wood *Senior Lecturer in Biostatistics, Department of Mathematics and Health Sciences and Clinical Evaluation, University of York*

Foreword

I find it an extraordinary experience that, as a Professor of Surgery, I have been asked to write the Foreword to a book, the subject of which six years ago, I would have thought of minimal relevance to my work, and of whose authors I had barely heard. This request is, however, an indication of a quiet revolution that has taken place in the British National Health Service. It is a revolution that has led to an unprecedented meeting of minds between clinicians and those academics of many disciplines who collectively can be grouped together as health service researchers. Such has been the coming together that I now believe, perhaps somewhat optimistically, that the majority of my clinical colleagues realise that it is no longer possible to practise safe and effective clinical medicine without input from those in the list of contributors to this book and their colleagues.

It is now a decade since the House of Lords Committee on Science and Technology drew attention to the fact that much of the research being funded by the National Health Service was biomedical in nature and not addressing the research needs of the Health Service, for example, in the field of evaluation of the clinical and cost effectiveness of new technologies. Their report led to the founding of the NHS Research and Development initiative, a venture which is undoubtedly turning out to be seen, worldwide, as one of the most significant and influential developments in the broad field of medical research.

The Research and Development initiative represents a swing of the research funding pendulum towards the answering of the questions faced daily by those of us with the task of delivering modern effective health care to the people of the United Kingdom from within a limited budget.

Past experience has shown that all too often the promise of new technologies developed by our basic science colleagues in university and pharmaceutical company laboratories has not materialised in the field. As Figure 19.1 on page 216 in this book demonstrates, for a product of basic research to be effective in practice it has to go through many phases before its benefits can be realised. Health Technology Assessment is now recognised as being one such phase and it is increasingly being accepted that it is necessary to ask about innovations *does this work, for whom, at what cost?*

As the Research and Development initiative has grown, and the largely unknown areas of Health Services Research in general and Health Technology Assessment in particular have developed, so it has become apparent that the research methods required for evaluation of the impact and effectiveness of new technologies need to evolve. It was obvious at the start of the Health Technology Assessment programme some 6 years ago that if it was to be successful, investment in developing the research methodologies was a priority. Consequently, the Methodology Panel of the Standing Group on Health Technology has become one of the most important and productive advisory panels which has underpinned the work of the whole of the R and D Programme.

This book represents the concerted efforts of a dedicated group of health services researchers who, with great industry, have developed and brought together for the first time the research methods used in Health Technology Assessment. This exercise has been supported by the *British Medical Journal* and the result is a concise, highly-readable explanation of the sophisticated technique used in the evaluation of new and existing technologies.

In the past there were many who looked somewhat scornfully at this type of research regarding it as not *real science*. How wrong they have been. Anyone who reads this book must realise that however sophisticated a laboratory finding, however much heralded as a breakthrough by the Press, it will come to nothing if it cannot be evaluated in the environment in which it has to be used. From now on those venturing into this area of research will have a concise, but authoritative statement of the methods used.

SIR MILES IRVING
*Professor of Surgery and
Director of NHS Health Technology Programme*

1 Researching health services

ANDREW STEVENS, RUAIRIDH MILNE AND
NICK BLACK

How should health care interventions (whether they be drugs, devices, procedures, settings of care, or even health care systems) be evaluated? What methods will best combine accuracy, speed, cheapness, feasibility, and usefulness? What are the limitations of the methods we use at the moment? Questions like these matter not just to researchers but also to patients, managers, and clinicians. If we do not know how best to assess the advantages and disadvantages of treatments, their cost, and their impact, then informed judgements – about individual treatment choices and about societal rationing decisions – are impossible.

This book is about these methods. It summarises the findings of 21 of the first reviews of methodological topics commissioned by the British National Health Service (NHS) Health Technology Assessment Programme.[1] This programme of reviews is the largest, most wide-ranging enterprise of its kind ever undertaken. The principal aim of this book is to provide a state-of-the-art guide to many of the key methods used in health services research. More detailed and lengthier accounts of each of the reviews appear elsewhere. Our aim has been to provide an accessible account of the latest thinking about health services research methods for a wide range of health care practitioners, students, and researchers who are planning or are undertaking studies of health care.

The NHS health technology assessment programme

Health technology assessment (HTA) is the term used internationally for the evaluation of specific health care technologies where the aim is to produce evidence with clinical or policy

1

relevance. Its origin was in the United States, where in 1972 the Office of Technology Assessment was set up to report to Congress on the potential beneficial and harmful effects of (in the case of health care) medical interventions.[2] Health technology assessment programmes now exist in many countries, including the United Kingdom.[3] The origins of the UK HTA programme go back to 1988, when a House of Lords committee reviewed the state of biomedical research and concluded that there was an imbalance in the allocation of funds.[4] The bulk of research funding in the NHS was spent on basic science and clinical research, while very little went into health services research and in particular the evaluation of services.[5] The NHS responded to this report by launching a Research and Development strategy in 1991, to ensure a mechanism for both identifying research priorities and funding commissioned research.[6] The HTA programme was established in 1993 as part of the Research and Development strategy with a budget of some £5 million ($8 million) a year, to ensure that "high quality research information on the costs, effectiveness and broader impact of health technologies is produced in the most efficient way for those who use, manage and work in the NHS".[1]

The programme commissions research to address the needs of the health service. A central question it must address is "Which questions need research-based answers?" This is decided by first, identifying possible questions of importance (which most years generates 1500 potential topics) and second, prioritising these to decide the 60 most pressing researchable questions.

Prioritisation is undertaken annually by the Standing Group on Health Technologies assisted by a secretariat at the National Coordinating Centre for Health Technology Assessment and six advisory panels. Five of these panels consider the need for research in specific areas of health care:

- the acute sector
- primary and community care
- pharmaceuticals
- diagnostics and imaging, and
- population screening.

The sixth panel, concerned with methodological issues, is innovative, seen in no other national system, and is concerned with the methods of health services research: the "how" rather than the "what" of HTA. The panel comprises experienced health services researchers with backgrounds in statistics, economics, epidemiology, clinical sciences, sociology, and health policy. The HTA programme is therefore playing a major part internationally in generating answers to important questions about the design and conduct of health services research.

The generation of needs-led methodological research

By 1998 the programme had funded reviews of 46 methodological topics, reports of which are now becoming available. Short accounts of the first 21 reviews are included in this book. These reviews have been through a five-stage process:

1. About 50 potential topics are identified each year by consultation with researchers and others.
2. The identified topics are prioritised by the Methodology Panel and the Standing Group on Health Technology, drawing on the expertise of their members and supported by *vignettes* prepared by their secretariat. Vignettes are briefing papers, describing the background to the topic, the extent to which existing methodological research has shed light on it, and possible ways forward.
3. The prioritised topics are advertised and researchers are invited to tender. Responses are judged both on quality and relevance (to the identified question) by a Commissioning Board, on which methodologists are strongly represented. Topics identified often have their focus narrowed or modified at this stage.
4. Research progress is monitored by the secretariat, for timeliness, value for money, and relevance to the commissioning brief.
5. Finally, reports are communicated to potential users through publication of articles in peer-reviewed journals and through the production of a peer-reviewed monograph series (Health Technology Assessment), available free to those in the public sector in the UK and accessible electronically over the World Wide Web. This book represents another, complementary form of dissemination.

Carrying out the reviews

Three major issues arise from the findings of these reviews. The first concerns the main conclusions which emerge from the five

3

principal strands of methodological research covered in this book.

- The development of generic outcome measures and patient-assessed outcomes will continue apace, reflecting as they do a growing concern with the appropriateness of health care to patients, and with the need to compare the costs and benefits of services.
- The range of methods available and needed for evaluating interventions extends well beyond randomised trials through non-randomised quantitative studies to qualitative methods.
- Statistical analysis is becoming more sophisticated in the light of the demands of new study designs and the appeal of Bayesian approaches.
- Secondary research, in which primary studies of different types are synthesised to enhance their value to clinicians and other health service decision makers, is now a major activity.

The value of all these developments is dependent both on the early identification of key health care technologies and on effective methods to communicate and implement the findings – and these also require appropriate methods.

The second issue concerns how to undertake reviews of methodological topics. Four principal methods were used by the reviewers:

- systematic reviews of the literature, which summarise not only empirical findings but also ideas;
- re-analysis of existing empirical work;
- other forms of primary research, particularly surveys of practitioners; and
- expert and group consensus, particularly for informed deduction, such as in setting out typologies of data sources, frameworks, and approaches.

The third and final issue concerns the return on investment in methodological research. The research presented in this book represents a considerable investment of resources which could be used for other types of research or direct patient care. It is right, therefore, that methodologists should pay attention to two key issues: Is it still worth spending money on developing methods for health services research? and, if so, is the programme going about it the right way? Although there has been some exploratory work in the UK seeking to assess the pay-back from health services research,[7] it has not looked at the even more demanding issue of pay-back from methodological research. In addition, could the identification and prioritisation of topics be done in a more logical or efficient way? And how sensitive is the current system of prioritising to the needs of both those doing health services research and those using them? These questions need to be addressed regularly to ensure that the research and development strategy achieves its maximum potential.

An outline of the book

All the review groups who have written the chapters that follow encountered the same two problems:

1. The systematic literature review, i.e. a review following a clearly documented approach, often needed to be supplemented or even replaced by the other approaches described above – the analysis of empirical work, surveys, and consensus views of experts.
2. Reviewers found a particular problem with the concept of systematicity when reviewing methodological work.

Discussions of the philosophical or theoretical aspects of systematicity and of the practicalities of strategies used for searching the literature appear in the Appendices.

The book is structured around five themes:

- measurement
- methods of evaluating health care
- statistical methods
- assessing, interpreting, and synthesising evidence, and
- ways of improving the evaluation and implementation of research findings.

Measurement

There is increasingly wide recognition of the need to assess outcomes from the patient's, as well as the professional's perspective. In Chapter 2, ways of assessing and comparing the attributes of existing instruments or questionnaires measuring health status and quality of life are discussed. Following on from that, if an evaluation intends to consider not only the effectiveness of an intervention but also its value or utility relative to other ways of spending health care funds, then a single index measure of the value of a person's state of health is needed. The advantages and disadvantages of the leading utility measures are considered in Chapter 3. Meanwhile, measurement of the costs of many interventions is far from straightforward. Which items to include, how to measure their use, and how to value them are discussed in Chapter 4. When the appropriate measures of benefits and costs have been selected, data have to be collected. Frequently this will be done by means of questionnaires to patients and health care staff, the design and use of which are considered in Chapter 5.

Methods of evaluating health care

Regardless of the method chosen, when evaluating health care we want to achieve high internal and external validity by minimising biases (including confounding). A fundamental decision is whether or not to adopt a design in which patients are randomly allocated to their intervention. The consequences of this decision are explored in Chapters 6 and 7 by means of a review of previous comparisons of the results of randomised and non-randomised studies and some new case studies. These enabled the reviewers to compare the size of any therapeutic effect obtained by each approach.

Despite the potential and, in many instances, actual advantages of randomised designs, the number of high quality RCTs is limited. The reasons for this state of affairs are considered in Chapter 8. One set of reasons covers ethical obstacles concerning the degree of uncertainty about an intervention's value that needs to exist, consent procedures, and interim analyses, and stopping rules (Chapter 9). Another, previously rather neglected, set of objections relate to the cultural or socioeconomic status of people. Our knowledge of these influences are reviewed in Chapter 10.

While many interventions can, in principle, be evaluated using a conventional trial design (whether randomised or not), this is not true of all. Some interventions are implemented at an organisational level (such as a new information technology strategy) or over a geographical area (such as a health promotion strategy). Evaluation of such interventions present several methodological problems. Approaches to dealing with them are discussed in Chapter 11. Important aspects of some interventions (such as a change of management style) cannot sensibly be evaluated using only quantitative methods. In such circumstances, qualitative methods may be more appropriate and productive (Chapter 12). In addition, qualitative methods are often needed in combination with quantitative approaches, such as in ensuring appropriate data are collected, and in understanding and interpreting the results.

Statistical methods

Whichever study design is adopted, quantitative methods require appropriate and good statistical principles to be employed. In Chapter 13 existing guidance on statistical methods is reviewed; recent and current developments are identified; and the frequency with which guidelines are used in practice is assessed. Most evaluative research employs "classical" or "frequentist" methods, with little use made of the Bayesian approach. In Chapter 14 the value of the latter approach, in which explicit quantitative use is made of external evidence in the design, monitoring, analysis, interpretation, and reporting of a study, is reviewed.

With the increasing importance of chronic illnesses, statistical methods that can deal not only with survival or quality of life but with both in combination, are needed. Statistical responses to this challenge are discussed in Chapter 15.

Assessing, interpreting, and synthesising evidence

The need for secondary research to obtain an overview of all the existing primary research findings is now well-established. While considerable attention has been paid to assessing the quality of randomised trials, less concern has been shown about economic evaluations. In Chapter 16 the quality of reporting such studies is appraised so that the amount of subjectivity in interpreting results is reduced.

A second issue concerns whether the results of different studies should be combined statistically and how should it be done. In Chapter 17 the considerable body of work in this area is reviewed, and methods available for combining study results are described. A third question is: What if anything, can be done to obtain an overview when there is insufficient clear, high quality research evidence? One option discussed in Chapter 18 is to employ a formal consensus development method to organise and synthesise a variety of forms of evidence.

Future improvements in managing evaluation

As will be clear from the above, there is considerable scope for improving our existing research methods and developing new techniques. At the same time, we can seek to improve the evaluation of health services in three other ways. First, we can try and identify new health care interventions before they become established. There is increasing interest in "horizon scanning" in which innovations are detected and thus subjected to evaluation, earlier in their development – an approach discussed in Chapter 19.

A second, related issue is that of determining the optimum time to evaluate a new intervention. At present there is no accepted formula for the timing of studies of new and fast-evolving technologies. Some possibilities for improving our performance in this area are considered in Chapter 20.

Thirdly, having evaluated an intervention, we need to improve the implementation of any research findings. The best methods for evaluating attempts at implementation are discussed in Chapter 21. We hope this book will help promote that implementation process.

Note

Copies of the full reviews on which the contributions to this book are based are available from: The NCCHTA, Mailpoint 728, Boldrewood, Southampton S016 7PX, UK; Fax +44 (0) 1703 595 639; email: hta@soton.ac.uk (free of charge to those working in the public sector in the UK). The full reviews may also be found on the World Wide Web: http://www.soton.ac.uk/~hta

References

1. National Coordinating Centre for Health Technology Assessment. *Identifying questions, finding answers. Annual report NHS Health Technology Assessment Programme 1997*, Leeds: NHS Executive, 1997.
2. US Congress, Office of Technology Assessment. *Identifying health technologies that work: searching for evidence*. OTA-H-608. Washington DC, US: Government Printing Office, September 1994.

3. Perry S, Gardner E, Thamer M. The status of health technology assessment worldwide. Results of an international survey. *Int J Technol Assess Health Care* 1997;**13**:81–98.
4. House of Lords Select Committee on Science and Technology. *Report Subcommittee II (Medical Research) Priorities in medical research*. London: HMSO, 1988.
5. Black NA. A national strategy for research and development: lessons from England. *Ann Rev Public Health* 1997;**18**:485–505.
6. Department of Health. *Research for health*. London: Department of Health, 1993.
7. Buxton M, Hanney S. How can pay-back from health services research be assessed? *J Health Serv Res Policy* 1996;**1**:35–43.

Part One
Measurement of benefits and costs

2 Patient-assessed outcome measures

RAY FITZPATRICK, CLAIRE DAVEY,
MARTIN J BUXTON AND DAVID R JONES

Increasingly research needs to assess outcomes of health care directly from the patient's perspective. This may be done by means of any of a vast array of questionnaires and interview schedules that we refer to here for reasons of simplicity as *patient-assessed outcome measures*. They are referred to by a variety of other terms in the literature, such as "quality of life", "health-related quality of life", "health status", "functional status", "subjective health status", or sometimes just "outcome measures". They have been developed to supplement mortality and conventional clinical, laboratory, radiological, and other measures of the outcomes of health care by direct assessment of matters of most concern to patients.

The main rationale for such measures is the fact that the majority of health care interventions have either as their primary or secondary purpose the improvement of one or more aspects of patients' health-related quality of life (Table 2.1). There is now extensive evidence that proxy reports of patients' health status and well-being such as those provided by health professionals or carers do not always agree with assessments patients make themselves.[1]

There are four principal applications of patient-assessed outcome measures:

1. They serve as measures of outcome in evaluative research. Their clearest role is in the randomised trial where potential biases in attributing changes in quality of life to interventions are minimised.
2. A second and related use is in audit and quality assurance.

Table 2.1   Dimensions of health-related quality of life assessed by patient-assessed outcome measures

Dimension	Illustrative content
I Physical function	Mobility, range of movement, physical activity Activities of daily living: ability to eat, wash, dress
II Symptoms	Pain, fatigue, nausea
III Global judgements of health	Global self-rating of health
IV Psychological well-being	Anxiety, depression, sense of control, self-esteem
V Social well-being	Family and intimate relations, social contact, integration, leisure activities
VI Cognitive functioning	Memory, alertness, ability to communicate
VII Role activities	Employment, financial concerns, household management
VIII Personal constructs	Satisfaction with bodily appearance, stigma, life satisfaction, spirituality
IX Satisfaction with care	Satisfaction with treatment, communication, interpersonal relations

3. They may be used in surveys to assess the health care needs of populations, either of geographical areas or of services such as attenders at a practice or clinic. This kind of use has provided additional evidence of, for example, social inequalities in health.[2] However, it is not yet clear whether patient-assessed outcome measures provide sufficiently clear and precise information about needs for particular services to be of use to planners.

4. The fourth application is to assist health professionals in individual patient care by providing a feasible and relevant set of information about patients' progress. To date, studies in which health professionals have been given additional information about their patients' progress by means of outcome measures have produced mixed results in terms of whether the quality of care was improved, although it is clear that patients believe such questionnaires provide information that is important for their doctor to know.[3]

The most important application, and the focus of this chapter, is therefore the use of patient-assessed outcome measures in evaluative research.

Nature of the evidence

There is now available an enormous array of patient-assessed outcome measures, differing in content, length, form of delivery, measurement properties, and intended purpose (Table 2.2). Whilst

Table 2.2   Different types of instruments and examples

Type of instrument	Example
Disease-specific	The Arthritis Impact Measurement Scales[4]
Site or region-specific	The Shoulder Rating Questionnaire[5]
Dimension-specific	McGill Pain Questionnaire[6]
Generic	SF-36[7]
Summary items	Question about limiting long-standing illness in the General Household Survey[8]
Individualised	Schedule for the Evaluation of Individual Quality of Life[9]
Utility	Health Utility Index[10]

there are several valuable guides to what is available, the investigator needs advice on considerations in selecting one or more instruments.[11,12] A systematic literature review was undertaken of the criteria that are required of patient-assessed outcome measures.[13] Literature discussing criteria for evaluating patient-assessed outcome measures was obtained by a combination of electronic searching of databases, hand-searching of selected journals, and in-house sources. A draft version of the review, based on 391 key references was submitted to 10 external consultants with diverse expertise in outcome measurement, and revised in the light of their comments and 18 additional references.

Findings

Appropriateness

The first and most fundamental consideration in evaluating a potential outcome measure is to determine its appropriateness. For example, a trial of hip or knee replacement surgery would need to consider whether it requires measures of pain, mobility, and activities of daily living that are generic and provide assessments of broader aspects of patients' health status, or specific measures that focus on problems in relation to joints. The sample size required would generally be larger and the interpretation different

15

if more generic measures were selected.[14] Several studies which have reviewed samples of randomised trials have reported that the majority of patient-assessed measures used were inappropriate.[15,16]

Reliability

There are two distinct but related aspects to reliability as a requirement of patient-assessed outcome measures. Firstly, the majority of measures assess any single construct, such as pain or social isolation, by means of several questionnaire items because several related observations are expected to produce a more reliable estimate than one. For this to be the case, items all need to be sufficiently homogeneous, that is all measuring aspects of a single construct. Thus questionnaire items intended to measure a single construct such as pain should have high internal consistency in that items should correlate adequately with each other. However, items of a scale should not be too homogeneous, because it is possible that the items are too similar and measure a very restricted aspect of, say, mobility.

The second aspect of reliability is the requirement that instruments yield the same results on repeated applications, assuming respondents' health status has not actually changed between measures. This property, reproducibility, is assessed by two administrations of a questionnaire between 2 and 14 days apart. Although the extent of association between scores is often assessed by correlation coefficients alone, further tests are needed to examine for overall shifts in the distribution of scores.[17]

Validity

In addressing whether an instrument is valid, that is whether it measures what it purports to measure, some methods of assessing validity cannot realistically be applied. In particular, criterion validity requires that we have available a "gold standard" measure against which a new instrument can be tested. This is rarely if ever the case and, were it the case, would minimise the need for a new measure.

Instead two broad and equally important approaches to validity have emerged in this field. On the one hand, qualitative judgements can be made about the range and content of items in a questionnaire. This approach, content validity, addresses whether the range of aspects of a phenomenon has been covered. For example, does a mobility scale contain items concerned with mobility in the home as well as in public spaces? Face validity addresses whether items appear, from their manifest expression, to measure what they purport to measure. These qualitative judgements can be structured in two ways. Most vitally, how extensive is the evidence that patients rather than experts participated in originally determining the content of an instrument? Secondly, patients, carers, and other relevant interests can participate in further testing the validity of an instrument to a new field of application.

The second broad approach is quantitatively to examine the construct validity of an instrument by examining patterns of relationships with a range of other variables. This does not depend on relationships with a single criterion variable. For example, we might expect poorer scores on a quality of life measure to be associated with greater disease severity, chronicity, poorer psychological mood, and more frequent utilisation of health services, all of course depending on details of the intended purpose of the measure and the health problem and intervention being considered.

Responsiveness

Responsiveness denotes, in this context, the extent to which an instrument is sensitive to changes over time that are of importance to patients. An instrument may provide reliable and valid information about aspects of patients' well-being but not be responsive. Guyatt and colleagues provide illustrative evidence of data from a randomised trial of chemotherapy for breast cancer in which, of four validated health status instruments completed by women, only one showed expected changes over time.[18]

Whilst responsiveness is increasingly accepted as a distinct and important requirement of a patient-assessed outcome measure, there is less agreement about how to assess it. Some studies have examined the degree of association of changes in the instrument of concern with changes over time in other parameters such as disease severity.[19] Other approaches identify as responsive those instruments that produce the largest amount of change when change is, for independent reasons such as the known effectiveness of an intervention, expected to occur.[20]

Precision

At one extreme on a spectrum of patient-assessed outcome measures are those that make a small number of simple and broad distinctions between health or quality of life states; at the opposite end are instruments that make many distinctions, most notably with continuous measures such as visual analogue scales. Unfortunately it cannot be argued that instruments that are capable of more distinctions are more precise. Elegant studies have shown that commonly used health status instruments may not equally represent the full underlying range of severity of problems. Stucki and colleagues, for example, argue from evidence with patients undergoing hip replacement surgery that the SF-36, one of the most frequently used measures, over-represents items of underlying moderate severity in physical disability in such a way that change scores can exaggerate improvement for respondents at that level of disability.[21] Ceiling and floor effects may also be a problem with instruments not being capable of measuring either improvement or deterioration beyond particular points on the instrument. Precision may be more apparent than real; for example a range of options from "1" to "4" is numerically transformed into 25%, 50% and so on.

Interpretability

Patient-assessed outcome measures produce numerical values that are not necessarily intuitively understandable. As patient-assessed outcome measures become more widely employed, repeated use will itself increase familiarity of the various audiences with the meaning of results. In addition, several different methods have been employed to increase interpretability. One approach is to correlate scores of such instruments with other information such as severe life events so that some commonsense or intuitive calibration of scores can be provided; a score of a particular magnitude on an instrument may, for example, be equivalent to the typical response to bereavement.[22] Another approach is to identify smallest clinically meaningful scores for an instrument by relating change scores for that instrument with independent judgements of the scale or clinical significance of such experiences.[23] To date interpretability is one of the least explored aspects of patient-assessed outcome measures.

18

Acceptability

It is essential that the burden to patients of completing outcome measures is minimised so that distress is as far as possible avoided and the refusal rate and rate of incomplete data for outcomes are reduced. In general terms the acceptability of patient-assessed outcome measures will be determined by their complexity, the distress arising from items, the overall layout, appearance and legibility of the questionnaire, and the time required to complete the task. Amongst patients who had undergone hip replacement surgery and were invited to return by post a 12-item questionnaire about hip pain and a 36-item generic questionnaire, the completion rate for the shorter instrument was 98% and for the longer instrument 73%.[24] It is useful to have available evidence about time to complete different instruments of the kind provided in one study: three patient-assessed outcome measures required 11, 18 and 22 minutes respectively.[25] Given the evidence that patients with poorer health status are less likely to complete quality of life measures, there is considerable risk of bias if this aspect is neglected.[26]

Feasibility

In addition to the possible burden to patients, it is necessary to estimate the likely impact of instruments on clinical staff and researchers in collecting, coding, and analysing patient-assessed data. At one extreme are brief self-completed questionnaires that impose minimal disruption; at the other extreme are instruments that require lengthy training of staff and lengthy interviews with patients to obtain data. Whilst investigators need to anticipate feasibility of data collection, they should not consider this a completely fixed property of instruments. Bernard and colleagues conducted a qualitative study of the collection of quality of life data from cancer patients in a randomised trial and concluded that staff attitudes to the value of such information were a key determinant of success in obtaining data.[27]

Recommendations

There are eight major criteria that investigators need to have in mind when selecting a patient-assessed outcome measure for an

Box 2.1 Questions that need to be addressed in selecting a patient-assessed outcome measure for use in an evaluative study

- Is the content of the instrument appropriate to the questions which the study trial is intended to address? (**Appropriateness**)
- Does the instrument produce results that are reproducible and internally consistent? (**Reliability**)
- Does the instrument measure what it claims to measure? (**Validity**)
- Does the instrument detect changes over time that matter to patients? (**Responsiveness**)
- How precise are the scores of the instrument? (**Precision**)
- How interpretable are the scores of the instrument (**Interpretability**)
- Is the instrument acceptable to patients? (**Acceptability**)
- Is the instrument easy to administer and process? (**Feasibility**)

evaluative study (Box 2.1). These criteria are not precisely defined in the literature and judgement is required to assess the evidence for any particular instrument. The properties of instruments, such as reliability and validity, are not fixed in some universal sense; strictly these are properties relative to a specific use. In selecting an instrument, investigators may have to trade-off criteria; an instrument that may have very substantial validity in collecting very detailed information about patients' experiences of an illness may not be acceptable and feasible.

Two kinds of developments are required in future research. Firstly, both from randomised and non-randomised studies in which patients complete more than one patient-assessed outcome instrument, measures can be directly compared so that more systematic evidence accrues of instruments' measurement properties. Secondly, researchers and clinicians should carry out reviews and assessments of particular widely used patient-assessed outcome measures in each health care field or specialty to help develop our understanding of the scope and appropriate methods for making the patient the primary judge of his or her outcome of care.

References

1. Sprangers M, Aaronson N. The role of health care providers and significant others in evaluating the quality of life of patients with chronic disease: a review. *J Clin Epidemiol* 1992;45:743–60.

2. Ahmad W, Kernohan E, Baker M. Influence of ethnicity and unemployment on the perceived health of a sample of general practice attenders. *Community Med* 1989;**11**:148–56.
3. Kazis L, Callahan L, Meenan R, Pincus T. Health status reports in the care of patients with rheumatoid arthritis. *J Clin Epidemiol* 1990;**43**:1242–53.
4. Meenan R. The AIMS approach to health status measurement: conceptual background and measurement properties. *J Rheumatol* 1982;**4**:785–8.
5. L'Insalata J, Warren R, Cohen S, Altchek D, Peterson M. A self administered questionnaire for assessment of symptoms and function of the shoulder. *J Bone Joint Surgery* 1997;**79A**:738–48.
6. Melzack R. The McGill Pain Questionnaire: major properties and scoring methods. *Pain* 1975;**1**:277–99.
7. Ware J, Sherbourne C. The MOS 36-item short-form health survey (SF-36). I. Conceptual framework and item selection. *Med Care* 1992;**30**:473–83.
8. Charlton J, Murphy M. Monitoring health: data sources and methods. In: Charlton J, Murphy M (eds) *The Health of Adult Britain 1841–1994*. London: The Stationery Office, 1997.
9. O'Boyle C, McGee H, Hickey A, O'Malley K, Joyce C. Individual quality of life in patients undergoing hip replacement. *Lancet* 1992;**339**:1088–91.
10. Torrance G, Furlong W, Feeny D, Boyle M. Multi-attribute preference functions: Health Utilities Index. *PharmacoEconomics* 1995;**7**:503–20.
11. Bowling A. *Measuring disease*. Buckingham: Open University Press, 1995.
12. McDowell I, Newell C. *Measuring health*. Oxford: Oxford University Press, 1996.
13. Fitzpatrick R, Davey C, Buxton M, Jones D. Evaluating patient-based outcome measures for use in clinical trials. *Health Technol Assess* (in press).
14. Dawson J, Fitzpatrick R, Murray D, Carr A. The problem of "noise" in monitoring patient-based outcomes: generic, disease-specific and site-specific instruments for total hip replacement. *J Health Serv Res Policy* 1996;**1**:224–31.
15. Guyatt G, Veldhuyzen Van Zanten S, Feeny D, Patrick D. Measuring quality of life in clinical trials: a taxonomy and review. *Can Med Assoc J* 1989;**140**:1441–8.
16. Gill T, Feinstein A. A critical appraisal of the quality of quality of life measurements. *JAMA* 1994;**272**:619–26.
17. Cox D, Fitzpatrick R, Fletcher A, Gore S, Spiegelhalter DJ, Jones DR. Quality of life assessment: can we keep it simple? *J Roy Statist Soc* 1992;**155**:353–93.
18. Guyatt G, Deyo R, Charlson M, Levine M, Mitchell A. Responsiveness and validity in health status measurement: a clarification. *J Clin Epidemiol* 1989;**42**:403–8.
19. Meenan R, Anderson J, Kazis L *et al.* Outcome assessment in clinical trials. Evidence for the sensitivity of a health status measure. *Arthritis Rheumatism* 1984;**27**:1344–52.
20. Liang M, Fossel A, Larson M. Comparisons of five health status instruments for orthopaedic evaluation. *Med Care* 1990;**28**:632–42.
21. Stucki G, Daltroy L, Katz J, Johannesson M, Liang M. Interpretation of change scores in ordinal clinical scales and health status measures: the whole may not equal the sum of the parts. *J Clin Epidemiol* 1996;**49**:711–17.
22. Testa M, Simonson D. Assessment of quality of life outcomes. *New Engl J Med* 1996;**334**:835–40.
23. Juniper E, Guyatt G, Willan A, Griffith L. Determining a minimal important change in a disease-specific quality of life questionnaire. *J Clin Epidemiol* 1994;**47**:81–7.
24. Dawson J, Fitzpatrick R, Murray D, Carr A. Comparison of measures to assess outcomes in total hip replacement surgery. *Quality in Health Care* 1996;**5**:81–8.

21

25. Read J, Quinn R, Hoefer M. Measuring overall health: an evaluation of three important approaches. *J Chronic Dis* 1987;**40** (Suppl. 1):7S–26S.
26. Hopwood P, Stephens R, Machin D. Approaches to the analysis of quality of life data: experiences gained from a Medical Research Council lung cancer working party palliative care trial. *Qual Life Res* 1994;**3**:339–52.
27. Bernhard J, Gusset H, Hurny C. Quality of life assessment in cancer clinical trials: an intervention by itself? *Support Care Cancer* 1995;**3**:66–71.

3 The use of health-related quality of life measures in economic evaluation

JOHN BRAZIER AND MARK DEVERILL

It has become common practice for economic evaluations to be conducted alongside randomised trials and other studies of effectiveness. An economic evaluation is the comparative assessment of the costs and effectiveness of health care interventions.[1] The purpose is to generate information that will assist decision-makers to determine the most efficient way of allocating their scarce resources between competing demands. Economic evaluation raises a host of methodological problems for researchers in the design of, data collection for, and analysis of studies.[2] This chapter is concerned with one set of problems, namely the assessment of effectiveness using measures of health-related quality of life (HRQoL). It addresses the question of how to judge the appropriateness of HRQoL measures for use in economic evaluation; it considers the limitations of measures that were not designed for use in economic evaluation, and it compares the five most commonly used economic measures of HRQoL (known as multi-attribute utility scales) used to generate quality adjusted life years (QALYs).

Nature of the evidence

Literature searches were undertaken of the topics identified. The core databases were MEDLINE, Embase, Science Citation Index, Social Citation Index, ECONLIT, and IBIS. The literature identified by these searches was extensive and included several thousand published articles.[3] Those found to be relevant to the questions addressed by the review provide the bases of what follows. The aim has been to synthesise the literature and to identify where there is consensus and disagreement.

Findings

Health-related quality of life measures

Measures of HRQoL are standardised questionnaires used to assess patient health across broad areas including symptoms, physical functioning, work and social activities, and mental well-being[4] (see example of the SF-36 health survey in Table 3.1). They consist of items covering one or more dimensions of health. They are either administered directly to patients, often by self-completion or less commonly through a third party (such as their doctor). Responses to items are combined into either a single index or a profile of several subindices of scores with the use of a scoring algorithm. For most measures this is typically a simple summation of coded responses to the items. The SF-36 physical functioning dimension, for example, has 10 items to which the patient can make one of three reponses: "limited a lot", "limited a little" or "not limited at all".[5,6] These responses are coded one, two, and three respectively, and the 10 coded responses are summed to provide a score from 10 to 30 (for the SF-36 these raw scores are transformed on to a 0–100 scale). A measure can be specific to a condition, such as the chronic respiratory questionnaire,[7] or general, such as the SF-36.

The patient focus of these measures has made them popular amongst health services researchers and clinicians for use in research (see Chapter 2). One of the questions addressed by this review is whether such measures can be used in economic evaluation, despite the fact that they have not been designed for the purpose.

Meanwhile, for economic evaluation, a small subset of measures of HRQoL have been specially developed, known as multi-attribute utility scales. These measures produce a single index score for each state of HRQoL from zero to one, where full health is equivalent to one and dead is zero. These single index scores, sometimes referred to by economists as health state utilities, are used to adjust

Table 3.1   An example of a measure of health-related quality of life – the SF-36 health survey[5]

Dimension	No. of items	Summary of content	No. of response choices	Range of response choice
Physical functioning	10	Extent to which health limits physical activities such as self-care, walking, climbing stairs, bending, lifting, and moderate and vigorous exercises	3	"Yes limited a lot" to "No, not limited at all"
Role limitations – Physical	4	Extent to which physical health interferes with work or other daily activities, including accomplishing less than wanted, limitations in the kind of activities, or difficulty in performing activities	2	Yes/No
Bodily pain	2	Intensity of pain and effect of pain on normal work, both inside and outside the home	5 & 6	"None" to "Very severe" & "Not at all" to "Extremely"
General health	5	Personal evaluation of health, including current health, health outlook, and resistance to illness	5	"All of the time" to "None of the time"
Vitality	4	Feeling energetic and full of life vs feeling tired and worn out	6	"All of the time" to "None of the time"
Social functioning	2	Extent to which physical health or emotional problems interfere with normal social activities	5 & 6	"Not at all" to "Extremely" & "All of the time" to "None of the time"
Role limitations – Emotional	3	Extent to which emotional problems interfere with work or other daily activities, including decreased time spent on activities, accomplishing less and not working as carefully as usual	2	Yes/No
Mental health	5	General mental health, including depression, anxiety, behavioural–emotional control, general positive affect	5 & 6	"All of the time" to "None of the time"

survival to calculate QALYs which can be used to assess the cost-effectiveness of interventions. The five most widely used are:

- Quality of Well-Being scale (QWB)[8]
- Rosser's disability/distress scale[9]

25

- the Health Utility Index version II and III[10]
- EQ–5D (EuroQoL[c])[11]
- 15–D.[12]

Table 3.2   Characteristics of multi-attribute utility scales

	Dimension	No. of levels per dimension	No. of health states	Method of estimating preference weights
Rosser	Disability	8	29	Magnitude
	Distress	4		estimation
QWB	Mobility, physical activity,		1170	Visual
	social functioning;	3		analogue scale
	27 symptoms/problems	2		
HUI-II	Sensory, mobility, emotion	4–5	240 000	Standard
	cognitive, self-care, pain,			gamble
	fertility	3		
HUI-III	Vision, hearing, speech	5–6	972 000	Standard
	ambulation, dexterity			gamble
	emotion, cognition, pain			
EQ-5D	Mobility, self-care, usual	3	243	Time trade-off
	activities, pain/discomfort,			and visual
	anxiety/depression			analogue scale
15-D	Mobility, vision, hearing,	4–5	Billions	Visual
	breathing, sleeping, eating,			analogue scale
	speech, elimination, usual			
	activities, mental function,			
	discomfort/symptoms,			
	depression, distress, vitality,			
	sexual activity			

The characteristics of these measures are summarised in Table 3.2. There is considerable overlap with other generic measures of HRQoL in terms of the dimensions that they cover. The crucial difference is the way they are scored. For all five measures, the weights have been obtained from a sample of the population to reflect their valuation of the different aspects of health. This review compares the performance of the five scales in terms of their practicality, reliability, and validity.[13,14]

Health economists have developed alternative methods for valuing the effects of health care. One is to generate QALYs from specially developed, condition-specific scenarios of health changes associated with each intervention.[15] Another is to ask people how much they are willing to pay for any benefits rather than to estimate QALYs.[16] However, only the multi-attribute utility scale method has been included in this review.

How to judge the appropriateness of health-related quality of life measures for use in economic evaluation

The psychometric criteria of practicality and reliability (in terms of stability) are necessary for any measure (see Chapter 2).[17] It is also essential to examine the validity of a measure, since there is little point in having a practical and reliable measure if it cannot be shown to be measuring the right concept. This is where the differences arise with conventional psychometric criteria. Economists are not seeking to measure or numerically describe patient health *per se*. What economists want to know is the *relative value* patients and others place on aspects of health in order to undertake more than the most rudimentary form of economic evaluation.[18,19] The value of any given improvement in health will be related to a change in HRQoL score, but these two concepts will not be perfectly correlated. For example, someone may regard a large improvement in health, such as the ability to walk upstairs, as being of little or no benefit if they live in a bungalow. Conversely, an apparently small reduction in pain may be highly valued by the patient. In economics, one test of validity would be its agreement with people's preferences revealed from making informed choices in a market setting.[20] However, for a number of reasons such situations do not arise in health care,[21] and therefore indirect ways have been used for assessing validity.

A three-part approach to examining validity may be adopted.[3] The first part is to examine the validity of the *description* of health, and second, the way items and dimensions of health are scored or *valued*. The descriptive validity of a measure concerns the comprehensiveness of its content, its suitability, and its sensitivity. There are a number of psychometric tests for assessing these aspects.[17] The scoring of a questionnaire should be based on the values people place on them rather than some arbitrary, if convenient, assumption of equal weighting. Economists have used a number of preference elicitation techniques for obtaining these weights and four of these are presented in Box 3.1. The techniques of standard gamble and time trade-off are preferred by economists over visual analogue scales and magnitude estimation because they confront the respondent with a choice.[13,22,23] In the case of standard gamble, for example, respondents are asked how much risk they would be prepared to take in order to avoid some poor health state.

Box 3.1 Techniques for eliciting values for health[13]

Visual analogue scale
"A typical rating scale consists of a line on a page with clearly defined endpoints. The most preferred health state is placed at one end of the line and the least preferred at the other end. The remaining health states are placed on the line between these two, in order of their preference, and such that the intervals or spacing between the placements correspond to the difference in preference as perceived by the subject" (p.18).

Magnitude estimation
"Here the subjects were asked to provide the ratio of undesirability of pairs of health states – for example, is one state two times worse, three times worse etc. compared to the other state? Then, if state B is judged to be x times worse than state A, the undesirability (disutility) of state B is x times as great as that of state A. By asking a series of questions all states can be related to each other on the undesirability scale" (p.25).

Standard gamble
"The subject is offered two alternatives. Alternative 1 is a treatment with two possible outcomes: either the patient is returned to normal health and lives for an additional t years (probability P), or the patient dies immediately (probability 1-P). Alternative 2 has the certain outcome of chronic state i for life (t years). Probability P is varied until the respondent is indifferent between the two alternatives, at which point the required preference value for state i is simply P; that is $hi = P$" (p.20).

Time trade-off
"The subject is offered two alternatives – alternative 1: state i for time t (life expectancy of an individual with the chronic condition) followed by death; and alternative 2: healthy for time $x < t$ followed by death. Time x is varied until the respondent is indifferent between the two alternatives, at which point the required preference value for state i is given by $hi = x/t$" (p.23).

A critical assessment of descriptive validity and the methods of valuation should help in understanding the extent to which a measure is able to be a valid measure of preferences. Together these two parts form theoretical validity. It is also important not to lose sight of *empirical validity*, and this forms the third part.

This can be tested indirectly in terms of convergence with stated preferences, such as the views of patients on the desirability of one state that they have experienced versus another, or hypothetical preferences where the researcher assumes one state would be preferred to another. A checklist of questions has been developed for these three aspects of validity, as well as reliability and practicality, which researchers are recommended to use when selecting a measure for use in economic evaluation (Box 3.2).[1]

Using health-related quality of life measures in economic evaluation which were not designed for the purpose

Measures of HRQoL, such as the SF-36 (Table 3.1), may have been found to be valid in a descriptive sense, but this does not necessarily mean that they are suitable for economic evaluation. The simple scoring algorithms used by most of these measures assume equal intervals between the response choices, and that the items are of equal importance. The SF-36 physical functioning dimension, for example, assumes that being limited in walking has the same importance as being limited in climbing flights of stairs, but there is no reason for this to be the case. For some measures the dimensions are combined into a single index by assuming equal weights, but such arbitrary scoring systems are unlikely to reflect people's preferences. These theoretical concerns have been confirmed by the evidence. A review of relevant studies revealed poor correlations between scores derived from measures of HRQoL based on simple scoring procedures and preference weighted measures.[2]

Many measures avoid the problems of combining dimension scores by reporting them separately as a profile. This presents problems when there are conflicts between the dimensions, such as in a study comparing surgical with non-invasive interventions, where surgery may be more effective at reducing symptoms but is associated with a range of complications. These measures also do not incorporate death as an outcome measure, and hence there is no easy solution where there is a conflict between the impact on survival and health-related quality between different interventions (see Chapter 15).

For these reasons, non-economic HRQoL measures have a limited role in economic evaluation. They can only be used to assess the *relative* efficiency of interventions where:

- one intervention is dominant (one intervention costs less and outcomes are superior);
- the interventions cost the same and outcomes are better on one dimension of the measure but no worse on any other or for any other outcomes, or outcomes are found to be identical and hence the comparison can be made in terms of costs (a cost-minimisation analysis).

It is impossible to assess relative efficiency when trade-offs must be made between dimensions of health or cost. In these circumstances, the results can be presented in a disaggregated form, but this may be of limited help to decision-makers given the difficulties in interpreting the scores. To overcome this problem we recommend that an economic measure of benefit, such as those described next, be used alongside a measure of HRQoL in studies intending to undertake an economic evaluation.

Comparing multi-attribute utility scales

The practicality, reliability, and validity of the five scales were assessed against the checklist using all published papers identified from a systematic search. There was little to choose between the instruments in terms of practicality and reliability. All measures are brief and easy to use, and four of them can be self-administered. The exception was the QWB, which has a lengthier interview schedule involving detailed probing of the respondents. There was some evidence of the test–re-test reliability of EQ-5D, 15-D, and HUI-III, although this has not been investigated adequately in any of the five measures.[3]

In terms of descriptive validity, the Rosser is inferior to the others in its coverage and has been shown to be less sensitive at detecting health differences than the EQ-5D.[24] The choice from the remaining four depends on the patient group being evaluated and views on the validity of including social aspects of health in the classification, since they differ considerably in their content. There was evidence of the ability of these measures to detect large differences between patient groups, but they also showed signs of insensitivity to smaller differences.[25] It was not possible to compare their descriptive validity owing to the different patient groups examined.

The QWB, Rosser, and the 15-D can be regarded as inferior to the other two measures because their values were obtained by

---

Box 3.2 Checklist for judging the merits of measures (components) of health-related quality of life for use in economic evaluation

- **Practicality**
  - How long does the instrument take to complete?
  - What is the response rate?
  - What is the completion rate?
- **Reliability**
  - What is the test–re-test reliability?
  - What are the implications for sample size?
  - What is the inter-rater reliability?
  - What is the reliability between places of administration?
- **Validity**
  - Description
    - Content validity:
      - Does the instrument cover all dimensions of health of interest?
      - Do the items appear sensitive enough?
    - Face validity:
      - Are the items relevant and appropriate for the population?
    - Construct validity:
      - Can the unscored classification of the instrument detect known or expected differences or changes in health?
  - Valuation
    - Do the assumptions about preferences seem credible?
      - What is the model of preferences being assumed?
      - What are the main assumptions of this model?
      - How well are the preferences of the patients/general population/decision-makers likely to conform to these assumptions?
    - Was the technique of valuation choice-based?
  - Quality of data
    - What are the background characteristics of the respondents to the valuation survey?
    - What was the degree of variation in the valuation survey?
    - Did respondents understand the valuation task?
    - What was the method of estimation (where relevant)?
    - Whose values have been used?
  - Empirical
    - Is there any evidence for the empirical validity of the instrument against:
      - Revealed preferences?
      - Stated preferences?
      - Hypothesised preferences?

31

methods not recognised by health economists as being valid techniques for eliciting patient preferences. The choice between HUI and the EQ-5D is less straightforward. They use different methods of eliciting weights (standard gamble and time trade-off respectively) and there is no consensus amongst health economists as to which is better. Furthermore, HUI weights are based on a Canadian sample and EQ-5D weights from a UK population. This dilemma is not resolved by evidence on empirical validity since this is so limited. For the HUI, there is a further choice between versions depending on whether the population are children (version II) or adults (version III).

The absence of published weights for HUI-III implies the EQ-5D is preferred for adult patients. This will have to be re-appraised when (Canadian) weights become available for the HUI-III. The jury is still out on the choice between these measures, and further comparative research is required. Empirical research may suggest, however, that neither is suitable for many patient groups, and that another measure, perhaps based on a more sensitive classification, is required. One solution would be to develop an entirely new multi-attribute utility scale.[26] Another is to obtain preference weights for a more sensitive measure of HRQoL.[27] Finally, a researcher may choose to estimate preferences for a specially developed, condition-specific scenario.

Recommendations

A researcher designing an economic evaluation alongside an effectiveness study should undertake a critical review of HRQoL measures for this purpose. We would recommend specifically that the checklist of questions referred to be used as guidance (Box 3.2). Researchers are encouraged to consider using either the EQ-5D or HUI (II or III depending on the age of the respondents) to supplement their chosen measure of HRQoL. Where these measures are inappropriate, other approaches to generating QALYs should be considered. This is a developing field and further research is required on the comparative performance of the HUI, EQ-5D, and other measures currently being developed.

References

1. Drummond MF, Stoddart GL, Torrance GW. *Methods for the economic evaluation of health care programmes.* Oxford: Oxford Medical Publications, 1987.

2. Drummond MF, Davies L. Economic analysis alongside clinical trials: revisiting the methodological issues. *Int J Technol Assess Health Care* 1991;7:561–73.

3. Brazier J, Deverill M, Harper R, Booth A. A review of the use of health status measures in economic evaluation. *Health Technol Assess* (in press).

4. Bowling A. *Measuring health: a review of quality of life and measurement scales.* Milton Keynes: Open University Press, 1991.

5. Ware JE, Snow KK, Kolinski M, Gandeck B. *SF-36 Health Survey manual and interpretation guide.* Boston, MA: The Health Institute, New England Medical Centre, 1993.

6. Brazier J, Harper R, Jones NMB *et al.* Validating the SF-36 health survey questionnaire: new outcome measure for primary care. *Br Med J* 1992;**305**: 160–4.

7. Guyatt GH, Thompson PJ, Bernam LB *et al.* How should we measure function in patients with chronic lung disease? *J Chronic Dis* 1985;**38**:517–24.

8. Kaplan RM, Anderson JP. A general health policy model: update and application. *Health Services Res* 1988;**23**:203–35.

9. Kind P, Rosser R, Williams A. Valuation of quality of life: some psychometric evidence. In: Jones-Lee MW (ed) *The value of life and safety.* North Holland, 1982.

10. Torrance GW, Furlong W, Feeny D, Boyle M. Multi-attribute preference functions. Health Utilities Index. *PharmacoEconomics* 1995;7:503–20.

11. Dolan P, Gudex C, Kind P, Williams A. *A social tariff for Euroqol: results from a UK general population survey.* Centre for Health Economics Discussion Paper 138, University of York, 1995.

12. Sintonen H. *The 15D measure of HRQoL: reliability, validity, and the sensitivity of its health state descriptive system.* NCFPE Working Paper 41, Monash University/The University of Melbourne, 1994.

13. Torrance GW. Measurement of health state utilities for economic appraisal: a review. *J Health Economics* 1986;5:1–30.

14. Williams A. Economics of coronary artery bypass grafting. *Br Med J* 1985;**291**: 326–9.

15. Cook J, Richardson J, Street A. A cost-utility analysis of treatment options for gallstone disease – methodological issues and results. *Health Economics* 1994; **3**:157–168.

16. Donaldson C, Shackley P, Abdalla M, Miedzybrozka Z. Willingness to pay for antenatal carrier screening for cystic fibrosis. *Health Economics* 1995;4:439.

17. Streiner DL, Norman GR. *Health Measurement Scales: a practical guide to their development and use.* Oxford: Oxford University Press, 1989.

18. Williams A. Measuring functioning and well-being, by Stewart and Ware. Review article. *Health Economics* 1992;**1**:255–8.

19. Culyer AJ. *Measuring health: lessons for Ontario.* Toronto: University of Toronto Press, 1978.

20. Johannesson M, Jonsson B, Karlson G. Outcome measurement in economic evaluation. *Health Economics* 1996;5:279–98.

21. Donaldson C, Gerard K. *Economics of health care financing: the visible hand.* London: Macmillan, 1993.

22. Richardson J. Cost-utility analysis – what should be measured. *Social Sci Medicine* 1994;**39**:7–21.

23. Nord E. The validity of a visual analogue scale in determining social utility weights for health states. *Int J Health Planning Manag* 1991;**6**:234–42.

24. Hollingworth W, Mackenzie R, Todd CJ, Dixon AK. Measuring changes in quality-of-life following magnetic-resonance-imaging of the knee – SF-36, Euroqol or Rosser index. *Qual Life Res* 1995;4:325–34.

25. Harper R, Brazier JE, Waterhouse JC, Walters S, Jones N, Howard P. A comparison of outcome measures for patients with chronic obstructive pulmonary disease in an outpatient setting. *Thorax* 1997;**52**:879–87.
26. Hawthorne G, Richardson J, Osborne R, McNeil H. *The Australian Quality of Life (AQoL) Instrument.* Monash University Working Paper 66, 1997.
27. Brazier JE, Usherwood TP, Harper R, Jones NMB, Thomas K. Deriving a preference based single index measure for health from the SF-36 *J Clin Epidemiol* (in press).

4 Collecting resource use data in clinical studies

KATHARINE JOHNSTON, MARTIN J BUXTON,
DAVID R JONES AND RAY FITZPATRICK

The increasing interest in performing economic evaluations alongside clinical studies has focused attention on a range of methodological concerns, both of principle and of best practice, in the process of obtaining and analysing data for costing purposes.[1] As the collection of economic data alongside clinical studies becomes routine, and decisions about data collection are made by investigators designing studies who may not themselves have experience or formal training in health economics, the importance of clarifying and, if possible, resolving these issues increases.

Clinical studies provide an opportunity to collect and analyse patient-specific resource use data. In principle this allows comprehensive and detailed data to be collected for each patient, but in practice there is a legitimate concern not to overburden the data collection process. Consequently, the choice of resource use items and methods for data collection need to be very carefully considered.

This chapter provides guidance on handling the key methodological issues. These issues include the types of cost to be included, sampling, data collection methods, as well as the analysis and presentation of the data.

Nature of the evidence

This chapter is based on a systematic review of existing reviews and applied studies. A number of statements of methods for

35

performing economic evaluation, both in general and in relation to randomised trials, are available.[2-5] These studies raise important issues of principle but they do not test empirically nor offer practical advice on handling these issues. Overall, the review found few examples of experimental studies testing the relative performance of different methods and thus many of the methodological issues remain untested.

Since methods for the collection and analysis of data for costing are still developing, there is a danger that further recommendations may impose rigid standards and constrain further methodological development. Some disagreement about how to handle particular issues is inevitable and, furthermore, resolution of many of the issues is, fundamentally, dependent on the theoretical perspective of the analyst, and the perspective of the study. When the status of methodological issues is discussed, the approach used is to identify a set of general issues where there is agreement, and to separate those issues where disagreement remains into those which reflect legitimate differences in values and perspective, and those more practical issues that are amenable to further elucidation by research.

Findings

In economic evaluation, cost is the product of two elements: the quantity of resources used and the unit costs used to value those resources. This chapter focuses on the former.

Types of cost

Costs can be classified into three broad categories: health service costs, non-health service costs, and other costs (Box 4.1). Health service costs include the direct costs of the intervention, such as hospital care, but may also include the direct costs associated with treatment for related and unrelated illnesses. An example of this distinction is presented in Box 4.2. For some interventions, future costs, the additional costs of treatment for diseases arising as a result of individuals living longer because of the initial intervention, may also be relevant.[6] A particular issue concerns study costs which, as well as referring to the costs of doing the research, are the costs of procedures in the study protocol that are required solely for the purposes of the study. The more pragmatic the study design, the fewer the costs that are protocol-driven, and the more

---

Box 4.1 Types of costs

- **Health service costs**
  - study costs
  - direct costs of the whole intervention
  - costs of treating other illnesses arising from the intervention
  - costs of treating illnesses unrelated to the intervention
  - future costs arising because individuals living longer because of the initial intervention
- **Non-health service costs**
  - costs incurred by other public sector budgets
  - informal care costs
  - patients' travel costs
  - other out of pocket expenses incurred by the patient
  - patients' time costs incurred in receiving treatment
  - productivity costs
  - future costs arising because individuals living longer because of the initial intervention
- **Other costs**
  - transfer payments

---

the resource use estimates are likely to reflect actual practice. Study costs can only be ignored if the resource use they represent is known not to affect outcome.[7–9]

Non-health service costs include the costs incurred by other budgets, such as social service costs and the costs of informal care. The sector incurring costs may change as budgetary arrangements change. Patients may incur non-health service costs including travel costs, other out of pocket expenses, and the time costs they incur when receiving treatment. Productivity costs may also be incurred by society and these include the costs, in terms of time and lost production, associated with the patient taking time off work. A final type of non-health service cost is future costs incurred, for example for food and shelter, as a result of longer survival because of the intervention.[6]

Other costs include transfer payments: flows of money from one group in society to another (such as social security benefits). Since they involve no resource consumption, they are usually excluded.[5]

Factors influencing the costs included

For each type of cost, a decision has to be made as to whether its inclusion is appropriate. This can be based on one or more of

Box 4.2 Example of types of health service costs

Study context

A randomised trial of cardiovascular screening and treatment led by nurses in general practices aimed to achieve a reduction in blood pressure, cholesterol concentration, and smoking prevalence among subjects in the intervention arm and thus reduce subsequent heart disease and stroke.

Types of cost

a) Study costs

Costs of research team and costs of any tests undertaken only for the purposes of the research.

b) Direct costs of the whole intervention

Programme costs (nurse time, consumables, buildings costs); drug costs; broader health service costs (health checks by doctors, other health checks); hospitalisations owing to heart disease.

c) Costs of treating other illnesses arising from the intervention

For example, where a visit to a practice nurse identified other illnesses for which treatment was required.

d) Costs of treating illnesses unrelated to the intervention

For example, inpatient costs for an unrelated accident.

e) Future costs arising from the longer survival resulting from the intervention

Costs of health care in added years of life.

Box 4.3 Potential factors influencing costs for inclusion

- Economic theory
- Perspective
- Form of economic evaluation
- Quantitative importance
- Attribution
- Time horizon
- Double counting

seven factors (Box 4.3). Some economists argue that economic welfare theory alone should dictate which costs are included.[10,11] The alternative, extra-welfarist position, is that the perspective of the decision-maker should influence the costs included.[12] The latter approach implies that a narrower range of costs will be included than the former. Possible perspectives of the study include the patient, the health service, or society. A health service perspective would imply that only health care costs are included. The form of economic evaluation to be conducted, such as cost-effectiveness analysis, or cost-utility analysis, may also determine the costs included. If the effects measured relate to health only, then it can be argued that costs should relate only to health.[13] This then relates back to the issue of perspective.

The expected quantitative importance of a type of cost should influence whether it is included. In principle, quantitative importance should be defined as the cost being large enough to have an impact on the cost-effectiveness ratio.[5] It may arise when resource use with a low unit cost occurs frequently or when resource use occurs infrequently but with a high unit cost. If there is no expected difference in the magnitude of a particular type of cost between two interventions being compared, then the cost could be excluded since it would not affect the choice between the interventions. Pre-trial modelling can be used to establish the expected quantitative effects of particular costs,[14] but what is regarded as quantitatively important is subjective, particularly when the magnitude of any difference in effect is not known.

A factor sometimes overlooked in the decision as to which costs to include is attribution: that is, whether resource use is attributable to the intervention. Determining attribution depends on having an understanding of the reasons why resources are consumed and having clearly defined criteria for attribution. Defining attribution according to the underlying clinical reasons for resource use is often arbitrary.[15-17] A pragmatic approach would be to present all costs as well as attempting to determine their attribution.

Double counting, that is counting the same cost twice or including an item both as a cost and as an effect, should be avoided.[18] For example, when including productivity costs, it is important not to count this as a societal cost and as a quality of life effect (see Chapter 2).

The time horizon, the period of time for which costs and effects are measured, may influence which costs are included. If a short time horizon is chosen, then long-term future costs would not be included. The time horizon chosen for the study also has implications for resource measurement since resource use may change over time or new resource items may be consumed,[19,20] ultimately affecting the direction and magnitude of cost differences.

Cost-generating events

Once the decision as to the types of costs to be included has been taken, it is necessary to identify the specific cost-generating events for which data collection is required. Examples of cost-generating events are a day in hospital or a visit to a doctor. If the key cost generating events can be established in advance, then it may be possible to limit data collection to these. Cost-generating events can be considered key where:

- the frequency of the event varies between the patient groups being compared or between patients within each group;
- the event has a large expected impact on total cost or the cost-effectiveness ratio.

Key cost-generating events can be identified from previous studies or pre-study data collection;[1] from pilot studies, models, or expert opinion.[14] All methods require having access to existing knowledge in the form of published studies or best available data.

Sampling

Sample size calculations require a judgement as to what constitutes an economically important difference to detect between patient groups in terms of cost-effectiveness, costs, or resource use. Existing information on the distribution and variability of cost-effectiveness, cost, or resource data is then required. Ideally, sample sizes would be calculated to estimate or test for differences in cost-effectiveness but this is technically difficult.[21] Instead, sample sizes can be calculated to estimate or test differences between costs. If data are unavailable to calculate sample sizes on costs, then sample sizes can be based on estimating or testing differences in an individual resource type, for example hospital days or doctor consultations.

In multicentre studies, a further sampling issue is the selection of centres.[22] A decision is also required as to whether to collect resource use data from all centres or a subsample.[23] If centres are likely to differ in terms of their economic characteristics, then it will be useful to collect resource use from all centres or to collect items of resource use that are likely to vary.

Data collection methods

Patient-specific resource use data can be collected from patients by one of the following methods:[24] interviews, questionnaires, case record forms, or diaries. Patient-specific resource use may also be obtained from existing records and administrative databases. In selecting a method of data collection from patients, potential sources of error to be addressed are non-response bias, evasive answer bias, selection bias, question format, and recall bias.[25] There is no clear evidence regarding the appropriate recall interval and recall has been shown to depend on the level of utilisation of resources, the frequency of use, type of resource, and severity of the illness. Studies comparing existing records and patients' reports have found the level of agreement to depend on the type of resource use. The incompleteness of records has been found to be problematic. An important practical issue is how easy existing records are to access or retrieve.[26]

The timing of data collection may be driven by: when the cost-generating events occur; when other data, such as quality of life, are to be collected; or when the study protocol events occur. The recall period also influences the timing of data collection.

Data analysis and presentation of results

Costs are calculated by multiplying resource use by the unit costs. Costs should be measured in a specific base year, adjusted for the effects of inflation and discounted so as to convert future costs into present values.

In synthesising cost data, issues such as how to pool the data and how to handle missing and censored data have to be addressed. Censored data is missing data arising because of loss to follow up, the presence of which has implications for the methods of analysis. Statistical approaches used to handle censored clinical data have been adapted for use with cost data.[27]

Uncertainty may arise from the data, the methods and the assumptions. The methods used to address uncertainty are statistical and sensitivity analyses, which have complementary roles.[5] Variability in cost data may be analysed using standard statistical methods but uncertainty in the cost-effectiveness ratio requires more complex methods which are still in development.[28] Sensitivity analysis involves the systematic investigation of how

41

changes in the selected assumptions affect the costs and cost-effectiveness (see Chapter 17).[29] It can be used to examine the impact of changes in, for example, length of stay, on total costs, or cost-effectiveness. It can also be used to generalise results.

The emphasis on reporting of studies should be on transparency: for example, presenting resource use and unit costs separately. Reporting of cost information should include sources of resource use and unit cost estimates, price bases, and discount rates.[30]

Recommendations

In undertaking studies, investigators should consider, in a systematic way, the various options for resource use data collection and ensure that the rationale for the chosen design is made explicit, and full use is made of existing evidence. The specific recommendations emanating from this review acknowledge two points. Firstly, methodological issues can be classified into different types:

- those where there is general agreement;
- those which remain open because of legitimate differences in values or perspectives;
- those amenable to further elucidation by empirical research (Table 4.1).

Issues categorised as remaining open can only be resolved by agreement as to what are the appropriate values and perspectives. Issues amenable to further research relate to the best ways of designing data collection exercises – the sources of information, the frequency of data collection, and modes of data collection. Thus, when designing studies, if investigators confront methodological options that are untested or unresolved, they should consider whether these could be formally investigated within the applied study.

Secondly, the dissemination of existing knowledge should be promoted since it can improve study design. For example, evidence on the distribution and variability of costs is required to estimate sample sizes. Similarly, information on the key cost generating events in other studies may inform the design of future studies. Performing pilot studies or conducting a period of pre-study data collection may also be useful.

Table 4.1   Status of methodological issues

Issues where there is agreement	Issues remaining open	Issues requiring further empirical research
Identifying perspective of study	Which perspective to adopt	Defining clear criteria for attribution of costs
Measure units of resource use and apply appropriate unit cost	Whether to adopt a welfare theoretic approach	Determining appropriate recall periods for data collection
Measurement of all health service costs	Whether to adopt an estimation or hypothesis testing approach	Exploring optimal sampling approaches
Need to use existing information or pre-trial study to inform study design		Sample sizes for cost-effectiveness
Use of sensitivity analysis		Issues surrounding multicentre trials and handling centre effects
Use of discounting		Investigation of methods of handling missing and censored data
Transparency in methods and results		Generalisability of resource use estimates

Those responsible for ensuring high standards of reporting of studies, for example journal editors, should ensure that authors are explicit about the perspectives adopted and methods used. They should also recognise that, given the limits on the length of published papers, authors may have to make such information available in technical reports.

Funding bodies should assist in the process of encouraging investigators to use existing data sets to inform design by the establishment of archives of data sets and should also actively encourage empirical testing of detailed methodological options within applied studies.

References

1. Drummond MF, Davies L. Economic analysis alongside clinical trials: revisiting the methodological issues. *Int J Technol Assess Health Care* 1991;7:561–73.
2. Drummond MF, O'Brien B, Stoddart GL, Torrance GW. Methods for the economic evaluation of health care programmes. 2nd edn. Oxford: Oxford University Press, 1997.
3. Drummond M. *Economic analysis alongside controlled trials*. Leeds: Department of Health, 1994.
4. Bulpitt CJ, Fletcher AE. Measuring costs and financial benefits in randomized controlled trials. *Am Heart J* 1990;119:766–71.
5. Gold MR, Siegel JE, Russell LB, Weinstein MC. *Cost-effectiveness in health and medicine*. New York: Oxford University Press, 1996.
6. Meltzer D. Accounting for future costs in medical cost-effectiveness analysis. *J Health Economics* 1997;16:33–64.
7. Rittenhouse B. *Uses of models in economic evaluations of medicines and other health technologies*. London: Office of Health Economics, 1996.
8. Canadian Coordinating Office for Health Technology Assessment. *Guidelines for economic evaluation of pharmaceuticals*. Ottawa: Canada, 1994.
9. Drummond MF, Jefferson TO, on behalf of the BMJ economic evaluation working party. Guidelines for authors and peer reviewers of economic submissions to the BMJ. *Br Med J* 1996;313:275–83.
10. Garber AM, Phelps CE. Economic foundations of cost-effectiveness analysis. *J Health Economics* 1997;16:1–31.
11. Birch S, Gafni A. Cost-effectiveness ratios: in a league of their own. *Health Policy* 1994;28:133–41.
12. Davidoff A, Powe NR. The role of perspective in defining measures for the economic evaluation of medical technology. *Int J Technol Assess Health Care* 1996;12:9–21.
13. Gerard K, Mooney G. QALY league tables: handle with care. *Health Economics* 1993;2:59–64.
14. Sculpher M, Drummond M, Buxton M. The iterative use of economic evaluation as part of the process of health technology assessment. *J Health Serv Res Policy* 1997;2:26–30.
15. Schulman KA, Glick H, Buxton M *et al.* The economic evaluation of the FIRST study: design of a prospective analysis alongside a multinational phase III clinical trial. *Controlled Clin Trials* 1996;17:304–15.

44

16. Hurley SF, Bond LM, Carlin JB, Evans DB, Kaldor JM. A method for estimating baseline health care costs. *J Epidemiol Community Health* 1995;**49**: 525–31.
17. Wonderling D, McDermott C, Buxton M *et al*. Costs and cost effectiveness of cardiovascular screening and intervention: the British family heart study. *Br Med J* 1996;**312**:1269–73.
18. Johannesson M. Avoiding double-counting in pharmacoeconomics studies. *PharmacoEconomics* 1997;**11**:385–8.
19. Jonsson B, Weinstein MC. Economic evaluation alongside multinational clinical trials: study considerations for GUSTO 11b. *Int J Technol Assess Health Care* 1997;**13**:49–58.
20. Dranove D. Measuring costs. In: Sloan FA (ed) *Valuing health care: cost, benefits and effectiveness of pharmaceuticals and other medical technologies*. Cambridge: Cambridge University Press, 1995.
21. O'Brien BJ, Drummond MF, Labelle RJ, Willan A. In search of power and significance: issues in the design and analysis of stochastic cost-effectiveness studies in health care. *Med Care* 1994;**32**:150–63.
22. Ellwein LB, Drummond MF. Economic analysis alongside clinical trials: bias in the assessment of economic outcomes. *Int J Technol Assess Health Care* 1996; **12**:691–7.
23. Menzin J, Oster G, Davies L *et al*. A multinational economic evaluation of rhDNase in the treatment of cystic fibrosis. *Int J Technol Assess Health Care* 1996;**12**:52–61.
24. Mauskopf J, Schulman K, Bell L, Glick H. A strategy for collecting pharmacoeconomic data during phase II/III clinical trials. *PharmacoEconomics* 1996;**9**:264–277.
25. Brown JB, Adams ME. Patients as reliable reporters of medical care process: recall of ambulatory encounter events. *Med Care* 1992;**30**:400–11.
26. Clark RE, Teague GB, Ricketts SK *et al*. Measuring resource use in economic evaluations: determining the social costs of mental illness. *J Mental Health Admin* 1994:32–41.
27. Fenn P, McGuire A, Phillips V, Backhouse M, Jones D. The analysis of censored treatment cost data in economic evaluation. *Med Care* 1995;**33**: 851–63.
28. Chaudhary MA, Stearns SC. Estimating confidence intervals for cost-effectiveness ratios: an example from a randomised trial. *Statist Med* 1996;**15**: 1447–58.
29. Briggs A, Sculpher M, Buxton M. Uncertainty in the economic evaluation of health care technologies: the role of sensitivity analysis. *Health Economics* 1994; **3**:95–104.
30. Mason J, Drummond M. Reporting guidelines for economic studies. *Health Economics* 1995;**4**:85–94.

5 Designing and using patient and staff questionnaires

ELAINE McCOLL, ANN JACOBY,
LOIS THOMAS, JENNIFER SOUTTER,
CLAIRE BAMFORD, ANDREW GARRATT,
EMMA HARVEY, ROGER THOMAS AND
JOHN BOND

In health services research, questionnaires are frequently the method of choice for gathering primary quantitative data from patients and health care professionals. The aim is to gather valid and reliable data from a representative sample of respondents. However, in common with other approaches to data collection, the information yielded by questionnaires is subject to error and bias from a range of sources. Close attention to issues of questionnaire design and survey administration can reduce these errors. However, many of the classic texts on questionnaire development, on which many researchers and health surveyors rely, are now quite dated[1,2] and most lack a scientific base, drawing instead on the accumulated experience and views of the authors.

Our aims in this chapter are to address this evidence gap by identifying established and innovative approaches to questionnaire design and administration, particularly those supported by evidence from experimental studies, and thereby to identify current best practice with respect to the design and conduct of surveys. The principal foci were:

- modes of questionnaire administration (face-to-face and telephone interviews; mailed and "captive audience" self-completion questionnaires; computer-assisted techniques);

- issues of question wording, choice of response formats, and question sequencing;
- issues of questionnaire formatting and other aspects of presentation; and
- techniques for enhancing response rates, with particular emphasis on mailed surveys.

We defined "questionnaire" to mean "structured schedules used to elicit predominantly quantitative information, by means of direct questions, from informants, either by self-completion or via interview".

Nature of the evidence

We were interested both in high grade evidence from comparative studies, and in lower grade evidence from descriptive studies and previous reviews, especially where higher grade evidence was lacking; we also sought information on the theoretical under-pinnings of survey response. We used the PsychLIT and MEDLINE databases as much of the innovative work on survey methods has been carried out in social and market research, rather than in the health sector; we searched for papers published between 1975 and 1996. Secondary references, cited in identified papers, were also obtained.

In synthesising our findings, we first reviewed "expert opinion" as expressed in the classic texts[1-3] and in papers on the theory of survey response, and then examined the identified evidence to see whether findings supported or refuted this conventional wisdom. With respect to many aspects of questionnaire design and administration, we found that evidence for the relative effectiveness of different approaches was scant. Moreover, we identified a number of limitations to the interpretation and applicability of the evidence. In particular, many comparative studies involved the manipulation of only one factor; yet as Dillman recognises, "the decision to respond (to a survey) is based on an overall, subjective evaluation of all the study elements visible to the prospective respondent".[2] We also recognised the existence of practical and ethical constraints in implementing some of the recommendations in a health setting.

Findings

Mode of administration

The two principal modes of questionnaire administration are self-completion by the respondent (traditionally this has been a pencil-and-paper exercise, but more recently computer presentation has been tried) or via an interviewer (either face-to-face or over the telephone; computers may be used for data capture). Expert opinion suggests that each mode has its advantages and disadvantages, as summarised in Table 5.1.

We identified six studies comparing face-to-face interviews with self-completion questionnaires. The two studies[4,5] which measured response rates reported significantly higher rates for interviews, while Cartwright also found that Asian women were under-represented in respondents to the mailed approach.[5] Five of the six studies[5-9] examined responses to sensitive questions; it is often asserted that the greater anonymity afforded by a self-completion questionnaire leads to greater honesty and that this approach is therefore more appropriate for surveys on sensitive or embarrassing topics. However, there was no clear evidence from these five studies that mailed survey subjects do respond more truthfully to questions on sensitive issues or make more critical or less socially acceptable answers than in an interview.

We also identified four studies in which telephone interviews were compared with mailed questionnaires; all were on health-related topics. Two of the studies found significantly higher response rates for the telephone approach,[4,10] and two found this approach cheaper.[4,11] One study reported a significantly higher response rate from the mailed questionnaire and a higher cost for the telephone survey; however, the rate of missing responses to individual questions was significantly higher in the mailed survey.[12]

In summary, evidence from the identified studies did not provide a consistent picture of the superiority of any one mode of questionnaire administration. In choosing a method, the researcher needs to consider trade-offs, for example between response rate and cost.

Question wording and sequencing

Most experts agree on general principles of question wording, as summarised in Box 5.1. We identified 11 studies on this issue,

---

Box 5.1 Principles of question wording[1,31]

- Use simple language; avoid acronyms, abbreviations, jargon and technical terms
- Keep the question short (i.e. sentence of less than 20 words approximately)
- Avoid questions which are insufficiently specific
- Avoid ambiguity
- Avoid vague words and those with more than one meaning (e.g. "dinner")
- Avoid double-barrelled questions (those with an "and" or an "or" in the wording)
- Avoid double negatives (e.g. a negative statement followed by a "disagree" response)
- Avoid proverbs and clichés when measuring attitudes
- Avoid leading questions (e.g. "Do you agree that the health service is underfunded?")
- Beware loaded words and concepts
- Beware of presuming questions
- Be cautious in use of hypothetical questions
- Do not overtax respondents' memories (e.g. by asking for detailed recall of trivial issues)
- Allow for "don't know" and "not applicable" responses if appropriate

---

though only two were on health-related topics. Evidence from these supported the notion that question wording and framing can have an important impact on the responses given. For example, Larsen *et al.* conducted two experiments on the use of quantifiers – verbal descriptors such as "often", "regularly", "sometimes" – in assessing symptom frequency; these words may be seen to be vague and different respondents may interpret them in different ways.[13] Findings showed that, while there were no statistically significant differences in the mean number of headaches reported, the quantifier "frequently" appeared to lead to under-reporting of this symptom.

Findings on whether a "don't know" category should be included were equivocal. Poe *et al.*, in a postal questionnaire containing only factual questions and sent to close relatives of recently deceased persons, found that the inclusion of a "don't know" option had no effect on overall response rates or item response rates, but that, for a quarter of the items in the questionnaire, the percentage of substantive replies (that is, endorsing one of the specific response

Table 5.1 Advantages and disadvantages of different modes of questionnaire administration

Mode of administration	Advantages	Disadvantages
Mailed self-completion	Cheaper than interviews No interviewer effects Greater anonymity for respondent Good for named individual and special population samples	Lower response rates than interviews – no-one to motivate respondent No control over response process (e.g. order in which questions are answered) Cannot ensure target recipient fills it in No opportunity to prompt or probe More errors in data Delay in getting back questionnaires through mail Not suitable for respondents with literacy problems
Supervised self-completion	Similar to mailed self-completion but interviewer/ researcher available to help and explain Can be used for groups More timely return of questionnaires vis-à-vis postal self-completion	Generally as for mailed self-completion and only suitable if target group of respondents comes together naturally
Face-to-face interviewing	Better for open-ended questions Flexible – interviewer can explain, probe and check Can have complex instructions and definitions High response rates – interviewer can motivate respondent Can use visual aids Can validate responses by observation	Interviewer may influence answers Inter-interviewer differences are a source of bias Other people may be present High cost

contd

Table 5.1 *contd*

Mode of administration	Advantages	Disadvantages
Telephone interviewing	Similar to face-to-face interviews Quicker than face-to-face interviews Cheaper than face-to-face interviews Greater anonymity for respondent Easier supervision and monitoring of interviewers	Coverage problems (those with no phone or ex-directory) Generally lower response rates than face-to-face interviews Less flexible than face-to-face interviews Cannot use visual aids Long interviews impractical Less intimate/poorer rapport Complex open-ended questions more difficult
Computer-assisted methods (questions presented on screen and answers entered directly into computer by interviewer or respondent)	Allows "tailoring" of questionnaire to individual respondent Extra step of data entry eliminated, thereby reducing costs Faster than traditional pencil-and-paper methods Improved data quality, since on-line data validation and editing possible Better control of fieldwork	High set-up costs Writing and testing questionnaire presentation/data capture program time consuming and error prone

categories) was significantly higher in the version without this option.[14] By contrast, Hawkins and Coney[15] and Bishop et al.[16] found that including a "don't know" option reduced the rate of uninformed response (that is, expressing a definite opinion on a fictitious matter) and concluded that offering such an option might reduce bias arising from a desire to appear knowledgeable or to hold a definite opinion.

Question ordering has received rather more attention. The conventional wisdom is that general questions should precede specific questions. Evidence from a number of studies supported this assertion. For example, Schuman et al.[17] found that general attitudinal questions (for example with respect to abortion) received significantly more positive endorsement when posed before a specific question on the same topic. Colasanto et al.,[18] in a study of HIV infection, looked at the effect of placing a question about whether HIV could be transmitted by donating blood before or after a question on transmission via blood transfusion. When the donation question was posed first, a significantly higher proportion thought it was possible to contract the disease through donating blood. It appeared that the question on blood transfusion, when it appeared first, helped to clarify the meaning of a potentially ambiguous question by means of a "contrast" effect and so reduced the number of erroneous responses.[19]

In summary, evidence from the identified studies generally supported the conventional wisdom on issues of question wording (though comparative studies were few), definition of response categories, and question sequencing.

Questionnaire appearance

Attention to the appearance of a questionnaire, including its length and layout, is important. As Sudman and Bradburn noted, in interview surveys, a well-designed questionnaire can simplify the tasks of both interviewers and data processors.[20] Through good design, the risk of errors in posing questions and coding responses can be reduced and potential variability between interviewers or coders can be minimised, thus reducing bias.

Evidence from comparative studies on aspects of questionnaire appearance was scant. However, we identified a number of papers outlining a theoretical basis to issues of design. Brown et al.[21] proposed a "task analysis" model of questionnaire response, based on social exchange theory,[22] which suggested that issues of questionnaire appearance can influence respondents' decisions at several stages. The first stage is arousal of interest in the task of questionnaire completion. The second stage is evaluation of the task, involving perceptions of the time and effort required to complete the questionnaire. The third stage is initiation and monitoring of the task of completion; here the actual burden of response becomes apparent. Appropriate design, in particular a layout that is clear, consistent, and uncluttered, can reduce the perceived and actual burden of response.

Jenkins and Dillman sought to develop a theory of self-administered questionnaire design, with particular emphasis on issues of format.[23] They emphasised the need for an understanding of "graphic non-verbal language", in other words the spatial arrangement of information and other visual phenomena such as colour and brightness. Drawing on theories of cognition, perception, and pattern recognition/processing, they argued for the need for consistency in the presentation of visual information, and derived five principles of design for self-administered questionnaires (Box 5.2).

Box 5.2 Principles of questionnaire design[23]

1. Use the visual elements of brightness, colour, shape and location in a consistent manner to define the desired navigational path for respondents to follow when answering the questionnaire.
2. When established format conventions are changed in the midst of a questionnaire, prominent visual guides should be used to redirect respondents.
3. Place directions where they are to be used and where they can be seen.
4. Present information in a manner that does not require respondents to connect information from separate locations in order to comprehend it.
5. Ask people to answer only one question at a time.

Enhancing response rates

In any survey a high response rate is desirable, since it increases the precision with which underlying population values can be estimated from sample results. In addition, a high response rate reduces the risk of bias; respondents are typically different from non-respondents in many respects – they are generally better motivated and more interested in the topic, are usually better educated, and the age and ethnic mix is often different (the very elderly and people from minority ethnic groups tend to be under-represented).[5,25,26]

The theory of social exchange postulates that the actions of individuals are influenced by the rewards they expect to get from completing these actions and the costs of doing so.[22] This suggests that many factors combine to influence the decision of a recipient of a questionnaire to respond. Potential respondents must have both the means to complete the questionnaire and the will to do so; the perceived costs of responding must not exceed the benefits of doing so. Many primary studies and reviews have addressed factors influencing the decision and ability to respond; most have focused on overall response rates, but the time to respond, response bias, and cost of the survey have also been considered by some authors.

In their review, Heberlein and Baumgartner showed that "saliency" – the apparent relevance, importance, and interest of the survey to the respondent – was the single most important factor affecting response rates.[24] Perhaps surprisingly, length of questionnaire appears to be less important; they found no significant first order correlations between length and response, although on controlling for saliency, longer questionnaires had poorer response rates. Health-related surveys, however, are likely to be seen as salient by the respondents, an assertion borne out by the findings of Cartwright[25] and Jacoby[26] who found no significant effect of length of questionnaire on response rates.

The number of contacts made with sampled individuals is another powerful factor in influencing response rates. Some researchers advocate prenotification, so that the recipients are primed for the arrival of the questionnaire. Linsky reported that prenotification significantly increased response rates.[27] However, Heberlein and Baumgartner demonstrated no advantage of advance contacts after controlling for total number of contacts, including reminders.[24] Almost all experts in survey design recommend the use of reminders. For example, Linsky showed that follow-up almost invariably increased response rate and that postcard reminders were as effective as letters.[27] Heberlein and Baumgartner showed that the first follow-up netted an additional return of 20%

of the initial sample, while second and third follow-ups brought in an extra 12% and 10% respectively.[24]

Other factors which have been shown to influence response rates include making a self-interest/utility appeal to the respondent, the use of incentives, and the type and rate of postage used (for example, higher response rates are generally demonstrated for stamped mail by comparison with franked or reply-paid envelopes). Perhaps surprisingly, anonymity (exclusion of any identifier, even a survey number) was shown to have no effect on initial response rates; or on item omission or completeness of response.[28,29] However, the use of numbered questionnaires (providing confidentiality rather than anonymity) was shown to boost overall response rates significantly, since targeted reminders could be used.

As already mentioned, a weakness of many of the studies we identified was that they sought to manipulate only one or two factors potentially influencing response rates; it is therefore difficult to interpret and generalise findings. In practice, the aim should be "to identify each aspect of the survey process that may influence either the quality or quantity of response and to shape each one of them in such a way that the best possible responses are obtained".[2] Moreover, few of the identified studies included an economic evaluation – for example, studies of the impact of reminders did not generally indicate whether the marginal benefit of the additional responses outweighed the marginal cost. Similarly, ethical considerations might preclude the application of some of the recommendations from social or market research in the health sector – for instance, postcard reminders might violate principles of confidentiality.

Recommendations

There can be no universal recommendations with respect to best practice in respect of questionnaire design and survey conduct. Rather, the researcher needs to take into account the aims of the study, the general study design, the population under investigation and the resources available. In a given study, trade-offs between the ideal and the possible are likely to be needed. However, some general principles can be stated.

- The principal objective should always be to collect reliable and valid data, in a timely manner, and within given cost and resource constraints, recognising that there may need to be a trade-off.

55

- In choosing a mode of questionnaire administration, consideration needs to be given to:
  - availability of an appropriate sampling frame
  - anticipated response rates
  - the potential for bias from sources other than non-response
  - the acceptability of candidate methods to respondents
  - the time available for data collection
  - the financial budget and
  - availability of other resources (such as skills and equipment).

While it may not be possible to quantify these parameters, some attempt should be made to estimate their relative magnitude for competing modes.

- In formulating questions and response categories, and in determining question order, researchers should bear in mind that survey respondents employ a wide range of cognitive processes in formulating their responses. To minimise bias and to reduce spurious inter-respondent variation, careful attention must be given to these issues. The established principles (Box 5.1) laid down in the traditional texts still hold good today.
- The task analysis model of Brown and colleagues[21] and the theory of social exchange[22] should underpin decisions regarding the physical design of questionnaires, as well as strategies for delivering and returning them. The aim should be to enhance the perceived and actual benefits of responding and to minimise the perceived and real costs.
- The saliency of the survey to respondents is a key factor in effecting high response rates; fortunately, surveys on health-related topics are likely to be viewed as relevant, important, and interesting. The perceived benefits of responding can also be enhanced by emphasising the self-interest/utility (rather than the altruistic) aspects of participating in the survey.
- The perceived and actual burden of responding can be reduced through appropriate question wording and an attractive questionnaire design and layout, drawing on the principles presented in Box 5.2. The aim should be to make the task of interpreting the questions and providing responses as easy as possible.
- Strategies for reducing the monetary cost to respondents include the use of prepaid and addressed envelopes for returning completed questionnaires (a must in mailed surveys). Financial

incentives are often offered in social and market research as token compensation for the time required to complete a questionnaire; however, such incentives are generally regarded as unethical in health research, and grant-awarding bodies tend to disapprove of the practice.[30]

- Above all, careful piloting and testing of draft versions of any questionnaire with the appropriate population is a vital step in questionnaire development. Questioning of respondents can indicate problems of comprehension. Analysis of responses can show whether all reasonable and relevant alternatives are included in response categories for closed questions. Data from the pilot study can also indicate the likely rate of response and inform sample size calculations for the main survey.

References

1. Moser CA, Kalton G. *Survey methods in social investigation.* London: Gower, 1971.
2. Dillman DA. *Mail and telephone surveys – the total design method.* New York: John Wiley & Sons Inc., 1978.
3. Fink A. (ed.) *The survey kit.* Thousand Oaks: Sage, 1995.
4. Hinkle AL, King GD. A comparison of three survey methods to obtain data for community mental health program planning. *Am J Community Psychol* 1978;6:389–97.
5. Cartwright A. Interviews or postal questionnaires? Comparisons of data about women's experiences with maternity services. *Milbank Quart* 1988;66:172–89.
6. Newton RR, Prensky D, Schuessler K. Form effect in the measurement of feeling states. *Social Sci Res* 1982;11:301–17.
7. Nederhof AJ. Visibility of response as a mediating factor in equity research. *J Social Psychol* 1984;122:211–15.
8. Oei TI, Zwart FM. The assessment of life events: self-administered questionnaire versus interview. *J Affective Disorders* 1986;10:185–90.
9. Boekeloo BO, Schiavo L, Rabin DL, Conlon RT, Jordan CS, Mundt DJ. Self-reports of HIV risk factors by patients at a sexually transmitted disease clinic: audio vs written questionnaires. *Am J Public Health* 1994;84:754–60.
10. Talley JE, Barrow JC, Fulkerson KF, Moore CA. Conducting a needs assessment of university psychological services: a campaign of telephone and mail strategies. *J Am Coll Health* 1983;32:101–3.
11. Pederson LL, Baskerville JC, Ashley MJ, Lefcoe NM. Comparison of mail questionnaire and telephone interview as data gathering strategies in a survey of attitudes toward restrictions on cigarette smoking. *Can J Public Health* 1994; 3:179–82.
12. McHorney CA, Kosinski M, Ware Jr JE. Comparisons of the costs and quality of norms for the SF-36 health survey collected by mail versus telephone interview: results from a national survey. *Med Care* 1994;32:551–67.
13. Larsen JD, Mascharka C, Toronski C. Does the wording of the question change the number of headaches people report on a health questionnaire? *Psycholog Record* 1987;3:423–7.

14. Poe GS, Seeman I, McLaughlin J, Mehl E. "Don't know" boxes in factual questions in a mail questionnaire: effects on level and quality of response. *Public Opinion Quart* 1988;**52**:212–22.
15. Hawkins DI, Coney KA. Uninformed response error in survey research. *J Marketing Res* 1981;**18**:370–4.
16. Bishop GF, Tuchfarber AJ, Oldendick RW. Opinions on fictitious issues: the pressure to answer survey questions. *Public Opinion Quart* 1986;**50**:240–50.
17. Schuman H, Presser S, Ludwig J. Context effects on survey responses to questions about abortion. *Public Opinion Quart* 1981;**45**:216–23.
18. Colasanto D, Singer E, Rogers TF. Context effects on responses to questions about AIDS. *Public Opinion Quart* 1992;**56**:515–18.
19. Schuman H, Presser S. *Questions and answers in attitude surveys: experiments on question form, wording and context.* New York: Academic Press, 1981.
20. Sudman S, Bradburn NM. *Asking questions.* San Francisco: Jossey-Bass Publishers, 1981.
21. Brown TL, Decker DJ, Connelly NA. Response to mail surveys on resource-based recreation topics: a behavioral model and an empirical analysis. *Leisure Sciences* 1989;**11**:99–110.
22. Thibaut JW, Kelley HH. *The social psychology of groups.* New York: Wiley, 1959.
23. Jenkins CR, Dillman DA. Towards a theory of self-administered questionnaire design. In: Lyberg L, Biemer P, Collins M *et al.* (eds) *Survey measurement and process quality.* New York: John Wiley & Sons Inc., 1997.
24. Heberlein TA, Baumgartner R. Factors affecting response rates to mailed questionnaires: a quantitative analysis of the published literature. *Am Sociolog Rev* 1978;**43**:447–62.
25. Cartwright A. Some experiments with factors that might affect the response of mothers to a postal questionnaire. *Statist Med* 1986;**5**:607–17.
26. Jacoby A. Possible factors affecting response to postal questionnaires: findings from a study of general practitioner services. *J Public Health Med* 1990;**12**:131–5.
27. Linsky AS. Stimulating responses to mailed questionnaires: a review. *Public Opinion Quart* 1975;**39**:82–101.
28. Campbell MJ, Waters WE. Does anonymity increase response rate in postal questionnaire surveys about sensitive subjects? A randomised trial. *J Epidemiol Community Health* 1990;**4**:75–6.
29. McDaniel SW, Rao CP. An investigation of respondent anonymity's effect on mailed questionnaire response rate and quality. *J Market Res Soc* 1981;**23**:150–60.
30. Bowling A. *Research methods in health – investigating health and health services.* Buckingham: Open University Press, 1997.
31. Oppenheim AN. *Questionnaire design, interviewing and attitude measurement.* London: Pinter Publishers, 1992.

Part Two
Methods of evaluating health care

6 Choosing between randomised and non-randomised studies

MARTIN McKEE, ANNIE BRITTON,
NICK BLACK, KLIM McPHERSON,
COLIN SANDERSON AND CHRIS BAIN

For studies that compare health care interventions to be valid, they must produce results that are generalisable to other potential recipients (high external validity), and they must also estimate outcome effects that can be reliably attributed to the intervention (high internal validity).

Studies can be divided into those that involve randomisation of subjects between comparison groups and those that do not. Both designs suffer from potential threats to external and internal validity. The randomised controlled trial (RCT) is seen by many as the "gold standard", as it should ensure that subjects being compared differ only in their exposure to the intervention being considered. However, the RCT has been criticised, with some arguing that design features tend to exclude, either consciously or otherwise, many of those to whom the results will subsequently be applied. Furthermore, in unblinded randomised trials the outcome of treatment may be influenced by practitioners' and patients' preferences for one or other intervention, leading to an inaccurate estimate of benefit. In contrast, non-randomised studies (non-randomised trials, cohort studies, case-control studies), whilst typically being more inclusive, can suffer from selection bias, in that the subjects may be allocated to treatment according to their initial prognosis.

These issues have led to considerable debate, although on the basis of limited empirical evidence. This chapter reviews what is known about the importance of the potential threats to validity for both randomised and non-randomised studies.[1] The impact on the measured effect size of using alternative study designs that seek to overcome threats to internal validity is considered in Chapter 7.

Nature of the evidence

Examination of these issues focused on the threats to internal and external validity of evaluations of effectiveness as well as the strategies proposed to overcome them (Table 6.1). These factors

Table 6.1   Threats to the validity of evaluative research and possible solutions

	Threatening factors	Proposed solution
Internal validity	Allocation bias (risk of confounding)	Risk adjustment and sub group analysis (analysis)
	Patient preference	Preference arms or adjustment for preference (design)
External validity	Exclusions (eligibility criteria)	Expand inclusion criteria
	Non-participation (centres/practitioners)	Multicentre, pragmatic design
	Not-invited (practitioner preference or administrative oversight)	Encourage practitioners to invite all eligible patients
	Non-participation (patients)	Less rigorous consent procedures

act through their effect on the distribution of potential-to-benefit among different groups. This can be illustrated schematically (Figure 6.1). The reference patient population is defined by an envelope. At some point, a treatment threshold is reached above which the overall benefits of treatment outweigh the risks. These constitute those patients eligible for treatment. Some eligible subjects are, however, excluded or do not participate, so the study population becomes a progressively smaller subset of the reference population, raising the question of whether it is valid to apply results obtained from this subsample to the reference population. In the example shown the envelope is triangular, reflecting the common situation in which a small number of people have a large ability to benefit with larger numbers benefiting less. The envelope and the subgroups within it can take many shapes depending on the condition and intervention.

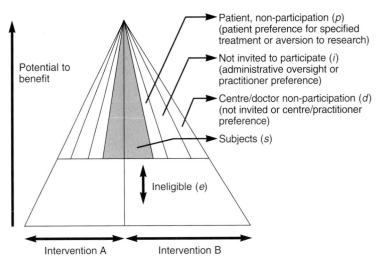

Patient, non-participation (*p*)
(patient preference for specified
treatment or aversion to research)

Not invited to participate (*i*)
(administrative oversight or
practitioner preference)

Centre/doctor non-participation (*d*)
(not invited or centre/practitioner
preference)

Subjects (*s*)

Potential to
benefit

Ineligible (*e*)

Intervention A   Intervention B

Figure 6.1   Schematic illustration of the relationship between subjects included in a study (shaded areas) and the reference population from which they are drawn in a study comparing two interventions, A and B.

The potential and actual importance of the factors that reduce the numbers included were explored through a series of systematic reviews examining four questions. Do non-randomised studies differ systematically from RCTs in the measured magnitude of treatment effect? Are there systematic differences between those included in or excluded from studies and do these influence the measured treatment effect? To what extent is it possible to overcome known or unknown baseline differences between groups that are not allocated randomly? How important are the preferences of subjects for an intervention and, if randomised to treatment that they would not choose, how does this affect their outcome?

In each case, papers addressing these issues were identified, such as those comparing the results obtained by different methods or those reporting the characteristics of those excluded or not participating. In addition, four case studies were undertaken, examining different types of intervention:

- coronary artery bypass grafting (CABG) and percutaneous transluminal coronary angioplasty (PTCA) (surgical);
- calcium antagonists (pharmacological);
- stroke units (organisational);
- malaria vaccines (preventive).

Findings

Comparing the results of RCTs and non-randomised studies

Eighteen papers were identified that directly compared the results of randomised and non-randomised studies,[2-19] in which the same intervention was investigated. Contrary to the view that non-randomised studies give larger estimates of treatment effects,[20-21] no obvious patterns emerge; neither RCTs nor non-randomised studies consistently give larger estimates of the treatment effect. Furthermore the type of intervention does not appear to be important. The four case studies indicate that, in addition to chance, there are several potential explanations for both larger and smaller estimates of treatment effects from RCTs than from non-randomised studies. The overall effect will reflect the relative importance of each issue in a particular case. A greater effect may be seen if those enrolled in a RCT receive higher quality care or are selected in such a way that they have a greater capacity to benefit than those in non-randomised studies. In contrast, there are several ways in which a RCT may produce a lower estimate of treatment effect.

- In non-randomised studies patients are typically allocated to a treatment that is considered most appropriate for their individual circumstances, such as the presence of co-existing disease. This may produce a larger treatment effect than in a randomised study in which such factors are disregarded.
- The design of a RCT or the decisions by practitioners to exclude certain individuals may create a sample with less capacity to benefit than in a non-randomised study.
- If those with strong preferences for a particular treatment show an enhanced response to treatment, this may not be captured in a blinded RCT, where subjects cannot express their preferences.
- Non-randomised studies of preventive interventions may include disproportionate numbers of individuals who, by virtue of their health-related behaviour, have greater capacity to benefit.
- Publication bias may be important if negative results are less likely to be published from non-randomised studies than from RCTs.

Although the evidence available is limited, the outcomes of non-randomised studies approximate to the results of RCTs when both use the same inclusion criteria and when potential prognostic factors are well understood, measured, and appropriately controlled in non-randomised studies (Box 6.1). The results of RCTs and of

---

Box 6.1 Different methods – different populations

Patients enrolled in the Beta Blocker Heart Attack Trial were compared with patients with a myocardial infarction who had been admitted to the Yale-New Haven Hospital and who met the criteria for entry to the trial in terms of age and primary diagnosis.[4] After adjustment for age and severity, the reduction in mortality with beta blockers at two years was lower among the trial subjects. However, when a subset of the Yale-New Haven patients was identified that met additional criteria for entry to the trial, such as indications strongly in favour of or against beta blockade, the outcome was similar to that in the trial, suggesting that the different initial result had been due to the inclusion of different types of patient.

---

non-randomised studies after adjustment are often not substantially different. Any variations are often no greater than those between different RCTs or between non-randomised studies. In our four case studies differences in effect sizes could have been due to chance, to differences in the populations studied, or to differences in the timing or nature of the intervention.

Do exclusions matter?

RCTs vary widely in the extent to which potential future recipients of treatment are included. The reasons cited for exclusion from trials may be clinical or scientific. Clinical reasons include subjects with a high risk of adverse effects, and belief that benefit has already been established for some groups or will be relatively small or absent. Scientific reasons include the ability to estimate the treatment effect with greater precision by having a relatively homogeneous sample[22] and reduction of bias by excluding those individuals most likely to be lost to follow-up.[23] In addition, many RCTs have blanket exclusions,[24] the reasons for which are often unstated, such as the elderly, women, and members of minority ethnic groups (Box 6.2).

Box 6.2 Exclusions – obvious and not so obvious effects

A review of 214 trials of the treatment for myocardial infarction published between 1960 and 1991 found that 61% formally excluded those aged over 75.[24] Examination of the age distribution of those studies with no formal exclusions suggested that this often happened but was unrecorded. Formal exclusions increased from 19% in the 1960s to 73% in the 1980s. One consequence was to exclude women disproportionately as they tend to have a later onset of coronary heart disease even though there are now more deaths from cardiovascular disease among women than men in the USA.

To overcome some of the perceived limitations of RCTs, some investigators have used large high quality clinical databases containing detailed information on patient prognostic factors. Patients identified from such databases tend to have a poorer prognosis than those included in randomised trials. When subjects are selected from such databases so as to meet the eligibility criteria used in RCTs, the treatment effect is similar in magnitude to that obtained from an RCT.[3,4]

High levels of exclusions can bring some benefits for the researcher such as increased precision of estimated treatment effects and reduced loss to follow-up. However, there are also some disadvantages such as the less certain extrapolation of results to other populations, the denial of effective treatment to those who might benefit, or the delay in obtaining definitive results because of the longer time required to recruit sufficient subjects.

Do differences in participation matter?

Most evaluative studies fail to document adequately the characteristics of those patients who, while eligible, do not participate. Such research is undertaken predominantly in university or teaching centres. Non-randomised studies are more likely than RCTs to include non-teaching centres, but it is not clear, on the basis of available evidence, how important this is. It is, however, plausible that such selective participation will exaggerate the measured treatment effect.

The effect of non-participation differs between RCTs which evaluate interventions designed to treat an existing condition and

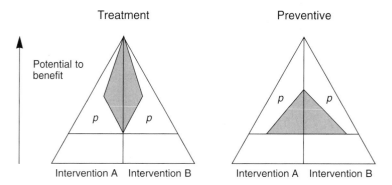

Figure 6.2   Schematic representation of possible differences in those participating in studies that evaluate treatments and those that evaluate preventive interventions.

those directed at preventing disease (Figure 6.2)[25]. Participants in RCTs evaluating treatments tend to be less affluent, less educated, and more severely ill than those who do not participate.[26] In contrast, those who participate in RCTs evaluating preventive interventions tend to be more affluent, better educated, and more likely to have adopted a healthy lifestyle than those who decline.[27] It is only possible to speculate about the consequences of this but it is plausible that low participation in RCTs of treatment may exaggerate treatment effects by including more skilful practitioners and subjects with a greater capacity to benefit, while RCTs of prevention may underestimate effects as participants have less capacity to benefit.

The impact of patient preference

Relatively little empirical research has been reported on the impact of an effect on outcome of patient preference. Only four studies have sought to measure preference effects [9,10,28,29] and they were either small or have yet to report full results (Box 6.3). In theory, preference could have an important impact on the results of RCTs, especially where the difference between treatments being compared is small. Such effects could account for some of the observed differences between results of RCTs and non-randomised studies. Methods have been proposed to detect preference effects reliably but while these approaches may contribute to our understanding of this phenomenon, none provides a complete answer.[30] This is

67

> ## Box 6.3 Patient's preferences and outcomes
>
> In a study of treatment for early breast cancer, 31 women were treated by surgeons favouring mastectomy, 120 by surgeons favouring breast conservation, and 118 by surgeons who were equivocal.[29] At 3 and 12 months, the last group, who were more able to express their own preferences, reported less anxiety and depression than the others. This may influence their final outcome after treatment.

mainly because randomisation between preferring a treatment or not is impossible and confounding may bias any observed comparison.

Is it possible to adjust for baseline differences between the arms of non-randomised studies?

Despite the evidence that the results of RCTs and non-randomised studies are often similar, differences in baseline prognostic factors clearly can be important. Absence of randomisation can produce groups that differ in important ways and it is necessary to consider whether it is possible to adjust for such differences. As it happened, in the four case studies, adjustment for imbalance in baseline prognostic factors between the arms of the non-randomised studies commonly changed the size of the measured treatment effect, but such changes were small and were not statistically significant. Furthermore, the direction of change was inconsistent. The limited ability to draw many conclusions from these case studies reflects both the lack of large randomised trials and that the outcomes were sometimes rare events. In the comparisons of CABG and PTCA, where the studies were large, there was evidence that the choice of treatment should be based on the patients' clinical features, with CABG better for some patients and PTCA for others. In this case, failure to undertake subgroup analysis or the use of a selected and thus atypical sample could give misleading results.

Overall, the evidence reviewed is very limited but suggests that differences in the populations studied by RCTs and non-randomised studies are likely to be of at least as much importance in explaining any differences as the issue of treatment allocation, and that if the two approaches are to be compared, this should only be done after subjects not meeting eligibility criteria for RCTs are excluded.

Recommendations

A large, inclusive, multicentre, fully blinded RCT, incorporating subgroup analysis is likely to provide the best possible evidence of effectiveness but there will always be circumstances in which randomisation is unnecessary, inappropriate, misleading, or impossible.[31] In those circumstances where there are genuine reasons for not randomising,[32] non-randomised studies can have a vital role in providing evidence. In such studies, adjustment for baseline imbalances should always be attempted, as rigorously and extensively as possible, and the procedures should be reported explicitly to assist readers' judgements. However, adjustment may not be sufficient if any important confounders remain unknown or unmeasurable.

Those conducting evaluative research (regardless of study design) must improve the quality of their reporting. Authors should define the population to whom they expect their results to be applied, what has been done to ensure that the study population is representative of this wider population, and any evidence of how it differs, the characteristics of those centres participating and any that declined, and the numbers and characteristics of those eligible to be included who either were not invited to do so or were invited and declined.

The findings have implications for the way in which evidence is interpreted. When faced with data from any source, using randomisation or not, it is important first to pursue alternative (non-causal) explanations thoroughly and examine the possible influence of chance, bias, and confounding, perhaps using sensitivity analysis where feasible. The generalisability to the population of interest should then be examined: was the range of practice settings and the study population representative of everyday practice?[7] Caution should be exercised where exclusions were for administrative convenience. Explanations should also be sought for lack of consistency in estimates of the magnitude of any effect between relevant studies.

When only non-randomised data are available, special consideration should be given to the potential for allocation bias and an assessment should be made of any attempts at risk or prognostic adjustment. In contrast, when only RCT evidence is found, especially if the trials are small, attention should be paid to the possible play of chance. The issues of generalisability and preference effects should also be considered. Ideally, to obtain an uncontaminated estimate of the physiological effect of a treatment, RCTs should be blind to all concerned but, for many interventions, this will be impossible. Also, the advantages of achieving high participation in RCTs should be balanced by the potential need for subgroup analysis. It should not be assumed that a summary result applies equally to all potential patients.

When both RCT and non-randomised studies have been conducted it is important to ascertain first whether subjects at similar risk experience a similar size of treatment effect. If they do, it may be reasonable to accept the broader range of effects likely to be present in the more inclusive non-randomised studies. Different results from RCTs and non-randomised studies cannot be assumed to be solely due to whether or not subjects were allocated randomly. Variations in the populations studied, in the characteristics of the intervention, and in the effect of patient preference appear equally likely explanations.

References

1. Britton A, McKee M, Black N, McPherson K, Sanderson C, Bain C. Choosing between randomised and non-randomised studies: a systematic review. *Health Technol Assess* (in press).
2. CASS Principal Investigators and their Associates. Coronary artery surgery study (CASS): a randomised trial of coronary artery bypass surgery. Comparability of entry characteristics and survival in randomised patients and nonrandomised patients meeting randomisation criteria. *JACC* 1984;**3**:114–28.
3. Hlatky MA, Califf RM, Harrell FE *et al*. Comparison of predictions based on observational data with the results of randomised controlled clinical trials of coronary artery bypass surgery. *JACC* 1988;**11**:237–45.
4. Horwitz RI, Viscoli CM, Clemens JD, Sadock RT. Developing improved observational methods for evaluating therapeutic effectiveness. *Am J Med* 1990; **89**:630–8.
5. Paradise JL, Bluestone CD, Bachman RZ *et al*. Efficacy of tonsillectomy for recurrent throat infection in severely affected children. Results of parallel randomised and nonrandomised clinical trials. *New Engl J Med* 1984;**310**: 674–83.
6. Paradise JL, Bluestone CD, Rogers KD *et al*. Efficacy of adenoidectomy for recurrent otitis media in children previously treated with tympanostomy-tube replacement. Results of parallel randomised and nonrandomised trials. *J Am Med Assoc* 1990; **263**:2066–73.
7. Schmoor C, Olschewski M, Schumacher M. Randomised and non-randomised patients in clinical trials: experiences with comprehensive cohort studies. *Statist Med* 1996;**15**: 236–71.
8. Yamamoto H, Hughes RW, Schroeder KW *et al*. Treatment esophageal stricture by eder-puestow or balloon dilators. A comparison between randomized and prospective nonrandomized trials. *Mayo Clin Proc* 1992;**67**:228–36.

9. McKay JR, Alterman AI, McLellan T, Snider EC, O'Brien CP. Effect of random versus nonrandom assignment in a comparison of inpatient and day hospital rehabilitation for male alcoholics. *J Consulting Clin Psychol* 1995;**63**: 70–8.

10. Nicolaides K, de Lourdes Brizot M, Patel F, Snijders R. Comparison of chorionic villus sampling and amniocentesis for fetal karyotyping at 10–13 weeks' gestation. *Lancet* 1994;**344**:435–9.

11. Emanuel EJ. Cost savings at the end of life. What do the data show? *J Am Med Assoc* 1996;**275**:1907–14.

12. Garenne M, Leroy O, Beau JP, Sene I. Efficacy of measles vaccines after controlling for exposure. *Am J Epidemiol* 1993:**138**:182–95.

13. Antman K, Amoto D, Wood W *et al*. Selection bias in clinical trials. *J Clin Oncol* 1985;**3**: 1142–7.

14. Shapiro CL, Recht A. Late effects of adjuvant therapy for breast cancer. *J Nat Cancer Inst Monographs* 1994, **16**: 101–12.

15. Jha P, Flather M, Lonn E *et al*. The antioxidants vitamins and cardiovascular disease – a critical review of epidemiological and clinical trial data. *Ann Intern Med* 1995;**123**:860–72

16. Pyorala S, Huttunen NP, Uhari M. A review and meta-analysis of hormonal treatment of cryptorchidism. *J Clin Endocrinol Metab* 1995; **80**:2795–9.

17. The Recurrent Miscarriage Immunotherapy Trialists Group. Worldwide collaborative observational study and meta-analysis on allogenic leukocyte immunotherapy for recurrent spontaneous abortion. *Am J Reprod Immunol* 1994;**32**:55–72.

18. Watson A, Vail A, Vandekerckhove P *et al*. A meta-analysis of the therapeutic role of oil soluble contrast media at hysterosalpingography: a surprising result? *Fertil Steril* 1994;**61**:470–7.

19. Reimold SC, Chalmers TC, Berlin JA, Antman EM. Assessment of the efficacy and safety of antiarrhythmic therapy for chronic atrial fibrillation: observations on the role of trial design and implications of drug-related mortality. *Am Heart J* 1992;**124**:924–32.

20. Colditz GA, Miller JN, Mosteller F. How study design affects outcomes in comparisons of therapy: I. Medical. *Statist Med* 1989;**8**:441–54.

21. Miller JN, Colditz GA, Mosteller F. How study design affects outcomes in comparisons of therapy: II. Surgical. *Statist Med* 1989;**8**:455–66.

22. Yusuf S, Held P, Teo KK. Selection of patients for randomized controlled trials: implications of wide or narrow eligibility criteria. *Statist Med* 1990;**9**: 73–86.

23. Haynes RB, Dantes R. Patient compliance and the conduct and interpretation of therapeutic trials. *Controlled Clin Trials* 1987;**8**:12–19.

24. Gurwitz JH, Nananda F, Avorn J. The exclusion of the elderly and women from clinical trials on acute myocardial infarction. *J Am Med Assoc* 1992;**268**: 1417–22.

25. Hunninghake DB, Darby CA, Probstfield JL. Recruitment experience in clinical trials: literature summary and annotated bibliography. *Controlled Clin Trials* 1987;**8**(Suppl.):6S–30S.

26. Barofsky I, Sugarbaker PH. Determinants of patients nonparticipation in randomised clinical trials for the treatment of sarcomas. *Cancer Clin Trials* 1979;**2**:237–49.

27. Davies G, Pyke S, Kinmouth AL. Effect of non-attenders on the potential of a primary care programme to reduce cardiovascular risk in the population. *Br Med J* 1994; **309**:1553–6.

28. Torgerson DJ, Klaber-Moffett J, Russell IT. Patient preferences in randomised trials: threat or opportunity. *J Health Serv Res Policy* 1996:**1**:194–7.

71

29. Fallowfield LJ, Hall A, Maguire GP, Baum M. Psychological outcomes of different treatment policies in women with early breast cancer outside a clinical trial. *Br Med J* 1990;**301**:575–80.
30. McPherson K, Britton AR, Wennberg JE. Are randomized controlled trials controlled? Patient preferences and unblind trials. *J Roy Soc Med* 1997;**90**: 652–6.
31. Black N. Why we need observational studies to evaluate the effectiveness of health care. *Br Med J* 1996;**312**:1215–18.
32. McPherson K. The Cochrane Lecture. The best and the enemy of the good: randomised controlled trials, uncertainty, and assessing the role of patient choice in medical decision making. *J Epidemiol Community Health* 1994;**48**: 6–15.

7 Comparisons of effect sizes derived from randomised and non-randomised studies

BARNABY C REEVES, RACHEL R MACLEHOSE,
IAN M HARVEY, TREVOR A SHELDON,
IAN T RUSSELL AND ANDREW MS BLACK

Randomised controlled trials (RCTs) are generally accepted as the "gold standard" method of evaluating the effectiveness of health care interventions,[1] but there are many circumstances in which RCTs are difficult to carry out, or are inappropriate.[2] There is considerable debate about the potential role of non-randomised designs (also referred to as quasi-experimental[3] and observational) for evaluating effectiveness. Health care decision makers need evidence about interventions which cannot readily be evaluated by RCTs as much as for those which can, but the findings of non-randomised studies may be biased and consequently lead to dangerous or wasteful decisions.[1,4]

Previous comparisons of estimates of effectiveness derived from randomised and non-randomised studies have suggested that the latter tend to report larger estimates of the benefit of the treatment being evaluated.[5-7] The perception that non-randomised estimates consistently favour new treatments has led to the assumption that discrepancies arise from bias. However, comparisons from the literature are often cited selectively. They may not have been carried out systematically and may have failed to consider alternative explanations for the discrepancies observed, such as differences in the populations, interventions, or outcomes studied (external validity), a greater susceptibility of non-randomised studies than

RCTs to publication bias, or a tendency for RCTs to underestimate effectiveness.[2]

The previous chapter focused on the ways in which contextual differences (external validity) between randomised and non-randomised studies can give rise to different estimates of effect size. This chapter complements the former by focusing on the internal validity of non-randomised estimates of effect size. We compare systematically estimates of effectiveness for specific interventions derived from randomised and non-randomised studies. Discrepancies attributable to bias and confounding are of primary interest, and we adopted two strategies to minimise the influence of differences in external validity:

1. We reviewed interventions for which randomised and non-randomised estimates of effectiveness were reported in a single paper, on the assumption that such papers were more likely to compare "like with like" than comparisons across papers.
2. We reviewed interventions for which the interventions, populations and outcomes studied were anticipated to be similar across studies and where randomised and non-randomised estimates of effectiveness were reported in different papers.

We also identified and classified study designs which have been proposed to overcome difficulties experienced with conventional RCTs.

Nature of the evidence

Studies comparing randomised and non-randomised estimates

Studies included:

- reviews which attempted to synthesise and compare primary data from a number of RCTs and non-randomised studies; [5,8,9]
- comprehensive cohort studies;[10-13]
- other studies in which primary data from randomised and non-randomised populations were compared (Box 7.1),[14-20] including those in which the non-randomised population received only one of the treatments compared in the RCT.[17-20]

Box 7.1 Study designs for comparing randomised and non-randomised evidence

A comprehensive cohort study consists of a cohort study of all subjects who are eligible for a RCT, with the subjects who participated in the RCT nested in the cohort.[22] Data for the randomised group are analysed conventionally. The whole cohort is analysed by epidemiological methods, with differences in prognostic factors between the randomised and non-randomised groups taken into account, to assess whether estimates of effect size are the same for the two groups. Schmoor *et al.* used this study design to compare mastectomy and breast preservation treatments, and other adjuvant treatments for breast cancer.[13]

Another example which compared randomised and non-randomised primary data is provided by Hlatky *et al.*[15] They compared the treatment effect of coronary artery bypass surgery vs medical treatment for coronary artery disease obtained using a non-randomised prospective database which included information about important prognostic factors, and three independent RCTs. Outcomes for medical and surgical patients in the prospective database, who would have been eligible for one of the RCTs, were analysed to provide a treatment effect which was then compared with the treatment effect found by the RCT. The three RCTs used different eligibility criteria, allowing the researchers to make three independent comparisons. In each case, the treatment effect estimated by the prospective database agreed well with the result of the RCT.

Two case studies

Two interventions were selected for review on the basis of the availability of estimates of effectiveness derived from different study designs and the homogeneity of the population studied, the intervention, and the outcome assessed: mammographic screening (MS) of women to reduce mortality from breast cancer, and folic acid supplementation (FAS) to prevent pregnancies affected by neural tube defects amongst women trying to conceive.

Findings

Studies comparing randomised and non-randomised estimates

Fourteen papers, reporting 38 comparisons between randomised and non-randomised findings, were identified. Three papers were reviews, [5,8,9] four were comprehensive cohort studies,[10-13] and seven compared primary data from RCTs and non-randomised populations indirectly.[14-20]

The "fairness" of the comparisons was assessed using a checklist of six items to identify the comparability of the randomised and non-randomised populations studied and the susceptibility of the comparisons to bias:

1. Were the same eligibility criteria used?
2. Were studies contemporaneous?
3. Was the assessment of outcome blinded?

Did the non-randomised estimates take account of confounding by:

4. Disease severity?
5. Comorbidity?
6. Other prognostic factors?

For each comparison, the items were scored as being satisfied or not by three assessors; 13 comparisons were classified as fair (>3/6) and 25 as unfair ($\leq$3/6).

Measures of the size of discrepancies between randomised and non-randomised estimates of effect size and the outcome frequency for intervention and control groups were calculated, where possible, for each comparison. Distributions of the size and direction of discrepancies were compared for fair and unfair comparisons. No analytic statistics were calculated because several papers included multiple comparisons and it was considered unlikely that comparisons within papers were statistically independent.

Discrepancies were much smaller for fair than unfair comparisons (Figure 7.1). For fair comparisons, there was no evidence that non-randomised estimates of effect size were more extreme than randomised ones. For unfair comparisons, there was a tendency for non-randomised estimates of effect size to be more extreme than randomised ones, which appeared more pronounced when considering comparisons based on larger sample sizes. The findings did not differ when only one comparison per paper was considered.

These results suggest that non-randomised estimates of effectiveness may be valid, if standard epidemiological methods of analysis (stratification or regression modelling) are used. The small size of the discrepancies between RCT and high quality non-randomised estimates also suggests that psychological factors, such as treatment

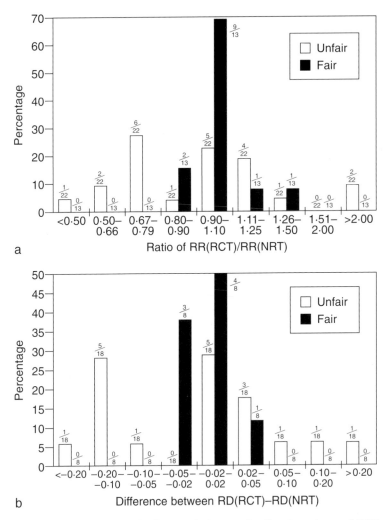

Figure 7.1 Distributions of the discrepancies between the effect size estimates of RCTs and non-randomised studies for fair and unfair comparisons: (a) ratios of RCT and non-randomised (NR) relative risks (RR) and (b) differences between RCT and non-randomised (NR) risk differences (RD).

preferences or willingness to be randomised, had a negligible effect on outcome. Previous comparisons may have overemphasised the differences between randomised and non-randomised estimates of effectiveness because of the poor quality of most non-randomised evidence.

We do not recommend generalising our results to other contexts for three main reasons:

1. Few papers were reviewed and our findings may depend on the specific interventions evaluated in these papers.
2. Most high quality comparisons studied randomised and non-randomised populations which met the same eligibility criteria; this may have had the effect of creating relatively uniform risk strata, reducing the possibility of confounding.
3. The papers which were reviewed may have been subject to some form of publication bias.

Authors are unlikely to have been disinterested about the comparison between randomised and non-randomised estimates, and findings appeared to support authors' viewpoints.

Two case studies

Thirty-four eligible papers were identified, 17 evaluating MS and 17 FAS.[21] For MS and FAS respectively, eight and four papers were RCTs, five and six were non-randomised trials or cohort studies, and three and six were matched or unmatched case-control studies; one MS and one FAS study used some other design.

Three reviewers used a detailed instrument to assess quality on four dimensions: reporting, the generalisability of the results, and the extent to which estimates of effectiveness may have been subject to bias or confounding. Both cohort and case-control studies had lower total quality scores than RCTs; cohort studies also had significantly lower scores than case-control studies.

Weighted regression analyses were used to investigate associations between effect size (relative risk) and various study characteristics. No effect of total quality was found after taking account of study design (Figure 7.2). Effect size estimates from RCTs and cohort studies were very similar, but case-control studies gave significantly different estimates for both MS (greater benefit) and FAS (less benefit). There are several reasons why case-control studies should give different estimates to RCTs and cohort studies. However, the inconsistency of the findings for MS and FAS suggests that the size and direction of the discrepancy is unpredictable and may be intervention-specific. Extreme caution should therefore be exercised when interpreting case-control estimates of effectiveness.

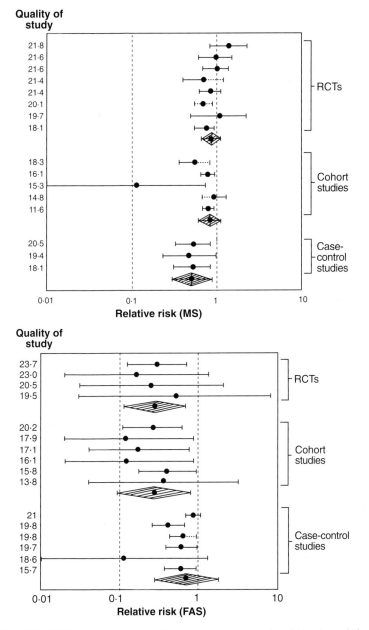

Figure 7.2   Blobbograms showing the effect size point estimates and confidence intervals for (a) MS and (b) FAS studies. Pooled estimates are shown separately for RCTs, cohort studies and case-control studies. Within each type of design, studies are ranked in order of quality.

79

We experienced difficulty using the instrument to measure quality and are doubtful about the validity of the scores obtained. Inter-rater agreement was modest for most instrument items. The internal consistency of different quality dimensions was poor, suggesting that the instrument had limited ability to discriminate the different dimensions; better internal consistency was found when the scores for all dimensions were pooled. Therefore, the lack of association between study quality and effect size could be due to any of the following:

- truly no association;
- inadequate assessment of quality, including the inability of the instrument to characterise different dimensions of quality which may have opposing influences; and
- heterogeneity of the intervention or population between studies, masking an association with quality, despite the choice of interventions anticipated to be relatively homogeneous.

Proposed solutions

Researchers have proposed designs to overcome a range of problems (Table 7.1), although the advantages have not always been substantiated. Ten study designs were identified, which were classified as "hybrids" if they were intended to provide both randomised and non-randomised estimates of effectiveness,[22-25] or as "RCT variants" if they adhered to the principle of randomisation but included some modification.[26-30]

Apart from the two-stage randomised trial design,[24] which has not been used, hybrid designs[22,23,25] assume that non-randomised estimates are unbiased, and that discrepancies between RCT and non-randomised estimates reflect the factors of interest, such as willingness to be randomised or treatment preference (Box 7.2).

The majority of RCT variants have been designed to overcome the problems of non-compliance and patient drop-out, either by excluding such patients[27,30] or by using time-to-a-request-for-open-treatment or drop-out as the study outcome.[29] These designs, therefore, promote measures of efficacy as opposed to effectiveness. Two other variants were identified, "response adaptive"[28] and "randomised consent"[26] designs (Box 7.3).

Attributing discrepancies between randomised and non-randomised estimates to factors such as patient preferences should not be assumed by default, since there may be residual confounding.

Table 7.1 Hybrid study designs and RCT variants and the issues which each is intended to address.

Study design	EXV	PTP	DRP	ENR	NTE	EFF	PEX	INC	CMP
Comprehensive cohort	●	●	●						●
Patient preference	●	●	●						●
Doctor preference			●						●
Two-stage trial	●	●	●	●	●				
Single randomised consent				●				●	
Double randomised consent				●				●	
Randomised "play the winner"							●		
Randomised discontinuation						●	●		●
Placebo run-in						●			●
Change-to-open label						●			●

Abbreviations:
EXV Designed to overcome the limited external validity that RCTs often have;
PTP Designed to accommodate patients' preferences for one or other of the treatments being compared;
DRP Designed to accommodate clinicians' preferences for one or other of the treatments being compared;
ENR Designed to encourage recruitment;
NTE Designed to estimate directly treatment and non-treatment effects, e.g. preference, willingness to be randomised;
EFF Leads to estimates of efficacy as opposed to effectiveness, by minimising drop-outs, non-compliance or crossover between treatments;
PEX Designed to minimise the exposure of patients to placebo;
INC Designed to overcome the problems of obtaining informed consent;
CMP Increases compliance.

Randomising patients prior to obtaining consent is likely to create as many problems as it solves, but may be a useful strategy when patients are likely to have a strong preference for an intervention. Other RCT variants may have a role when the aim is to measure efficacy.

Recommendations

Our aim was to establish "safety limits" for non-randomised studies of different levels of quality, that is the size of effect which would be unlikely to be explained by bias, in order to guide interpretation of non-randomised evidence. However, this aim was thwarted because the influence of variations in internal and external validity between studies could not be satisfactorily distinguished. High quality non-

Box 7.2 Hybrid designs

Comprehensive cohort studies (Box 7.1) and patient preference trials are the commonest hybrid designs. In a patient preference trial all eligible patients are asked whether they prefer one of the treatments being compared and, if a preference is expressed, they are allocated to the preferred treatment.[23] Patients who have no preferences for either treatment are randomly allocated to the treatments being compared and form a randomised group, which is analysed conventionally. The distinction between a comprehensive cohort and a preference trial is subtle, since preference for a treatment is often the reason for a patient refusing to participate in a RCT.

The patient preference trial was proposed for situations in which patients' preferences could affect the outcome of a study, exemplified by Henshaw *et al.*[32] who used the design to compare women's experiences of medical and surgical abortion. About half of the women expressed a preference for a particular treatment and half underwent randomisation to treatments. Women who received their preferred treatment found it highly acceptable, whereas surgical abortion was significantly more acceptable amongst women who were randomised.

Box 7.3 Response adaptive and randomised consent designs

A response adaptive design allocates patients to treatments randomly but with varying probability, depending on the outcomes for patients already treated;[28] a new recruit has a higher probability of being allocated to the treatment currently "doing best". It is intended to reduce the exposure of patients to the inferior treatment and to reach a conclusive answer more quickly, but both of these aims are disputed. There are also concerns about stopping rules and how best to analyse the data. The design is only feasible when the outcomes of treatment are known quickly enough to influence the allocation of new recruits.

Randomised consent designs randomise patients prior to obtaining consent,[26] and usually seek the consent of patients to their allocated treatment without disclosing the treatment comparison.[31] This strategy is intended to facilitate recruitment and to avoid patients' treatment preferences. The precise method of obtaining consent is crucial; disclosing the treatment comparison is likely to obviate the benefits of prior randomisation, but failing to do so may be unethical. Such studies underestimate differences in effectiveness, since patients who do not consent to their assigned treatment are nevertheless analysed in the groups to which they are randomised.

randomised studies appear to be valid, but we do not recommend generalising this finding to circumstances where randomised and non-randomised estimates are obtained from different populations, or where randomised estimates may not be available.

Most non-randomised studies reviewed were of poor quality. We strongly recommend, however, that the use of non-randomised designs to evaluate health care interventions should not be rejected on the basis of this evidence. Rather, there is a need for more evidence about the comparability of findings from RCTs and non-randomised studies with the use of comprehensive cohort studies. Ineligible patients who receive one or other of the treatments being investigated, not usually included in comprehensive cohorts, should also be followed up. These designs need to be used in areas where randomised trials are the preferred design, as well as areas where RCTs are problematic, in order to assess the generalisability of evidence about the validity of non-randomised evidence.

Data analyses should focus on using the RCT estimate of effectiveness, and estimates of the effect of other prognostic factors from the entire cohort, to predict outcome frequencies for different groups of non-randomised patients; close agreement between predicted and observed results would be strong evidence of the validity of non-randomised studies. However, this approach cannot take account of interactions between an intervention and prognostic factors.

Comprehensive cohort studies are expensive, since they need at least double the sample size of a conventional RCT. It would therefore be attractive to nest RCTs within established high quality prospective clinical databases, where relevant prognostic factors and outcomes are routinely recorded and where large numbers of patients can be studied at reasonable cost. Consideration also needs to be given to the optimal way of obtaining consent and offering randomisation or treatment choices to patients.

The approach adopted in the two case studies should not be pursued for other interventions until a more suitable instrument has been developed to assess different attributes of studies. The instrument must be able to assess all aspects of study design which may influence effect size and should make explicit the aspect that each item is intended to assess. Separate instruments are likely to be required for different study designs, necessitating some method of standardising quality scores when comparisons are made across study designs.

References

1. Peto R. Large scale randomized evidence: large simple trials and overview trials. *Ann N Y Acad Sci* 1993;**703**:314–40.
2. Black N. Why we need observational studies to evaluate the effectiveness of health care. *Br Med J* 1996;**312**:1215–18.
3. Cook TD, Campbell DT. *Quasi-experimentation design and analysis issues for field settings*. Boston: Houghton Mifflin, 1979.
4. Doll R. Doing more good than harm: the evaluation of health care interventions. *Ann N Y Acad Sci* 1993;**703**:313.
5. Chalmers TC, Matta RJ, Smith H, Kunzler AM. Evidence favouring the use of anticoagulants in the hospital phase of acute myocardial infarction. *New Engl J Med* 1977;**297**:1091–6.
6. Colditz GA, Miller JN, Mosteller F. How study design affects outcomes in comparisons of therapy: I. Medical. *Statist Med* 1989;**8**:441–54.
7. Miller JN, Colditz GA, Mosteller F. How study design affects outcomes in comparisons of therapy: II. Surgical. *Statist Med* 1989;**8**:455–66.
8. Reimold SC, Chalmers TC, Berlin JA, Antman EM. Assessment of the efficacy and safety of antiarrhythmic therapy for chronic atrial fibrillation: observations on the role of trial design and implications of drug-related mortality. *Am Heart J* 1992;**124**:924–32.
9. Wortman PM, Yeaton WH. Synthesis of results in controlled trials of coronary artery bypass graft surgery. In: Light R (ed.) *Evaluation studies review annual*, Vol 8. London: Sage Publications, 1983.
10. CASS principal investigators and their associates. Coronary artery surgery study (CASS): a randomised trial of coronary artery bypass surgery. Comparability of entry characteristics and survival in randomized and non-randomized patients meeting randomization criteria. *J Am Coll Cardiol* 1984;**3**:114–28.
11. Paradise JL, Bluestone CD, Bachman RZ *et al.* Efficacy of tonsillectomy for recurrent throat infection in severely affected children: results of parallel randomized and non randomized clinical trials. *New Engl J Med* 1984;**310**: 674–83.
12. Blichert-Toft M, Brincker H, Andersen JA *et al.* A Danish randomized trial comparing breast preserving therapy with mastectomy in mammary carcinoma. Preliminary results. *Acta Oncol* 1988;**27**:671–7.
13. Schmoor C, Olschewski M, Schumacher M. Randomized and non-randomized patients in clinical trials: experiences with comprehensive cohort studies. *Statist Med* 1996;**15**:263–71.
14. Gray-Donald K, Kramer MS. Causality inference in observational vs experimental studies. *Am J Epidemiol* 1988;**127**:885–92.
15. Hlatky MA, Facc MD, Califf RM *et al.* Comparison of predictions based on observational data with the results of RCT of coronary artery bypass surgery. *J Am Coll Cardiol* 1988;**11**:237–45.
16. Horwitz RI, Viscoli CM, Clemens JD, Sadock RT. Developing improved observational methods for evaluating therapeutic effectiveness. *Am J Med* 1990; **89**:630–8.
17. Kirke PN, Daly LE, Elwood JH, for the Irish Vitamin Study Group. A randomized trial of low dose folic acid to prevent NTD. *Arch Dis Child* 1992; **67**:1442–6.
18. Ward L, Fielding JWL, Dunn JA, Kelly KA, for the British Stomach Cancer Group. The selection of cases for randomised trials: a registry of concurrent trial and non-trial participants. *Br J Cancer* 1992;**66**:943–50.
19. Fisher B, Costantino JP, Redmond CK *et al.* Endometrial cancer in tamoxifen-treated breast cancer patients: findings from the National Surgical Adjuvant

Breast and Bowel Project (NSABP) B-14. *J Nat Cancer Inst* 1994;**86**:527–37.

20. Marubini E, Mariani L, Salvadori B *et al*. Results of a breast cancer surgery trial compared with observational data from routine practice. *Lancet* 1996;**347**: 1000–3.

21. MacLehose RR, Reeves BC, Harvey IM, Black AM, Sheldon TA, Russell IT. A review of randomised controlled trials, quasi-experimental and observational study designs for evaluating the effectiveness of health care. *Health Technol Assess* (in press).

22. Olschewski M, Scheurlen H. Comprehensive cohort study: an alternative to randomised consent design in a breast preservation trial. *Methods Information Med* 1985;**24**:131–4.

23. Brewin CR, Bradley C. Patient preferences and randomised clinical trials. *Br Med J* 1989;**299**:313–15.

24. Rucker G. A two-stage trial design for testing treatment, self-selection and treatment preference effects. *Statist Med* 1989;**8**:477–85.

25. Korn EL, Baumrind S. Randomised clinical trials with clinician preferred treatment. *Lancet* 1991;**337**:149–52.

26. Zelen M. A new design for randomized clinical trials. *New Engl J Med* 1979; **300**:1242–5.

27. Amery W, Dony J. A clinical trial design avoiding undue placebo treatment. *J Clin Pharmacol* 1975;**15**:674–9.

28. Rosenberger WF, Lachin JM. The use of response-adaptive designs in clinical trials. *Controlled Clin Trials* 1993;**14**:471–84.

29. Högel J, Walach H, Gaus W. Change-to-open label design: proposal and discussion of a new design for clinical parallel-group double-masked trials. *Arzneimittel Forsch* 1994;**14**:97–9.

30. Davis CE, Applegate WB, Gordon DJ, Curtis RC, McCormick M. An empirical evaluation of the placebo run-in. *Controlled Clin Trials* 1995; **16**:41–50.

31. Altman DG, Whitehead J, Parmar MKB *et al*. Randomised consent designs in cancer clinical trials. *Eur J Cancer* 1995;**31**:1934–44.

32. Henshaw RC, Naiji SA, Russell IT, Templeton AA. Comparison of medical abortion with surgical vacuum aspiration: women's preferences and acceptability of treatment. *Br Med J* 1993;**307**:714–17.

8 Factors that limit the number, quality, and progress of randomised trials

ROBIN J PRESCOTT, WILLIAM J GILLESPIE,
CARL E COUNSELL, ADRIAN M GRANT,
SUSAN ROSS, IAN T RUSSELL AND
SANDRA KIAUKA

The randomised controlled trial (RCT) is widely accepted as the most powerful research method for evaluating health technologies. Its principal strength is that it minimises bias (the risk of being misled by systematic errors), provided that a number of well-established principles are followed in the design and conduct of the study. Although these principles are now widely recognised and understood both by those responsible for decisions about policy and practice, and by clinical and health services researchers, there is little reliable information from randomised trials for most therapeutic activities. Some interventions pre-date the general acceptance of this method as the appropriate way to evaluate efficacy and effectiveness. Another reason for the dearth of reliable information is the failure, until recently, of health care systems to require up-to-date systematic reviews of research evidence. It will be some years before that situation changes. Further explanations lie in weaknesses in the design, conduct, and analysis of RCTs and in professional and public perceptions of the place of research within health care.

Nature of the evidence

Material for this review has come from a wide variety of sources. In an ideal world we would hope to see the randomised trial method applied to many aspects of the conduct of RCTs, to provide us with "gold standard" evidence. Unfortunately, such studies are uncommon and are limited to a few specific topics such as alternative methods of obtaining consent. For the main part, therefore, our evidence comes from a mixture of randomised trials, systematic reviews, surveys, and from statistical and economic theory.

We conducted a systematic review to assemble a comprehensive bibliography reporting factors limiting the number, progress or quality of randomised trials, to classify the bibliography as to the factors identified and the strength of information provided about these factors, and to collate and report the findings, identifying areas where firm conclusions can be drawn, and others where further research is required. In this chapter we summarise the results of that review, with particular emphasis on recommendations for good practice in RCTs.

Findings

We present our evidence under six headings: design, barriers to undertaking RCTs, conduct, analysis, reporting, and costs.

Design

The research question

A systematic review of existing research evidence should first be conducted to clarify the most timely and important question. A well-formulated research question should specify the participants (sampling frame), interventions, and outcomes. In patient selection, wide eligibility criteria are generally preferable to give representativeness and good recruitment rates. However, there may be advantages in a more homogeneous population when expensive or hazardous interventions are evaluated which might only be justified in high risk groups.[1] Outcome measures need to be clinically and socially relevant (that is, of importance to the patient), well-defined, valid, reliable, sensitive to clinically or socially important change, and measured at appropriate times in relation to the intervention and the natural history of the condition. There is evidence that the use of intermediate or surrogate outcomes has been common and frequently misleading (Box 8.1).[2]

Box 8.1 Intermediate outcomes may be misleading – an example

Fleming and DeMets'[2] report states:
"the use of surrogates recently produced misleading results in the setting of advanced colorectal cancer. The frequently used treatment of 5-fluorouracil in combination with leucovorin showed a statistically significant improvement in the complete response plus partial response rate (23%) compared with the improvement seen with 5-fluorouracil alone (11%). Despite this difference in tumour response, there was almost no difference in overall survival (relative risk 0.97). These results were taken from a meta-analysis of almost 1400 patients."

We examined the use of intermediate outcomes in two recently completed systematic reviews (Table 8.1).[3,4] Only one randomised trial of hormone replacement therapy reported outcomes of clinical importance. For vitamin D and its analogues, clinical outcomes were more frequently recorded. Most studies of hormone replacement therapy were carried out in women in the early post-menopausal period, in whom fractures would be infrequent in the

Table 8.1 The use of clinically important (fractures) and intermediate (bone mass) outcomes in two systematic reviews in osteoporosis

Theme	RCTs identified	Clinically important outcomes only (no. of participants)	Intermediate outcomes and clinically important outcomes (no. of participants)	Intermediate only (no. of participants)
Hormone replacement therapy in osteoporosis/ fracture prevention	33 (to end 1993)	None	A None B 1 (70)	32 (1390)
Vitamin D analogues in fracture prevention in the elderly	25 (to end 1995)	A 2 (176) B 3 (239)	A 4 (6020) (intermediate 576) B 8 (360)	8 (2144)

A Fracture event of which patient was aware; B Radiologically identified vertebral fracture.

short and medium term. In contrast, the majority of participants in the vitamin D studies were elderly and at higher risk of sustaining a fracture during a feasible study period.

Choice of study design

A fundamental choice is between a parallel group or a crossover design. The potential advantage of the latter is its efficiency as it requires fewer participants for the same power.[5,6] However, in many situations (for example, in surgery, obstetrics, psychotherapy) a crossover design is not possible. The simultaneous investigation of two or more treatments is efficiently approached by the use of a factorial structure within either parallel group or crossover designs. The use of factorial designs has been uncommon.[7] The simple parallel group design with a fixed sample size remains the most commonly used. It should not however be automatically adopted, as other designs can sometimes produce major benefits.

Avoiding bias

Protection from selection bias is provided by true random allocation, by secure concealment with the use of telephone or computer-based randomisation,[8] and by analysis based on the groups as allocated, thereby ensuring that the groups being compared differ only by chance. Performance bias can be minimised by blinding treatments (where possible) and by employing clearly described treatment policies, identical for each group apart from the intervention under examination. Detection bias may be avoided by arranging that the outcome is assessed in ignorance of the treatment allocated, and attrition bias by ensuring that systematic differences in withdrawals from the trial during follow-up are detected.

Sample size

The views of Fayers and Machin[9] are endorsed (Box 8.2). Funding bodies, independent protocol review bodies, ethics review panels, and journal editors should all demand provision of sample size calculations. These should consider a sensitivity analysis and give indicative estimates rather than unrealistically precise numbers. Small trials should be clearly reported as hypothesis forming.

Box 8.2 Recommendations concerning sample size (adapted from Fayers and Machin 1995)[9]

- Sample size calculations should always be made pre-study.
- Post-hoc power calculations should not be encouraged.
- Estimates of sample size should not be regarded as precise, because of uncertainty about the underlying assumptions.
- Nomograms give sufficient precision.
- A "sensitivity analysis" should show the effects of varying the initial requirements of the study.
- A small, underpowered, randomised trial is better than no study provided:
  - the results are presented as hypothesis forming;
  - the trial is registered before commencement.
- Report of sample size calculations should be demanded by:
  - funding bodies
  - independent protocol review committees
  - ethical review panels
  - journals to which reports are submitted.

Barriers

Barriers to clinician participation
To overcome the problems which are listed in Box 8.3, the study should address a question that is seen as important by clinicians. The protocol should be as clear and simple as possible, with the minimum required of clinicians, and straightforward data collection. Where possible, dedicated research staff should be available to support the research and provide encouragement to clinical staff. Pragmatic designs may be more acceptable to clinicians since this type of design permits more clinical freedom.

Barriers to patient participation
To overcome these barriers (Box 8.3), the demands of the study should be kept to a minimum consistent with its scientific purpose. The extent and purpose of the study and the investigations should be clearly explained. Patients should be supported in the difficult decision to take part in a randomised trial, and should not be placed under pressure to do so. Dedicated research staff may be required to help with providing information, obtaining patient consent, and monitoring the recruitment process.

Box 8.3 Main barriers to clinician and patient participation in randomised trials

- **Clinicians**
  - time constraints
  - limited staffing and training
  - inadequate rewards and recognition
  - adverse impact on the doctor/patient relationship
  - concern about extent of participation required by patients
  - mismatches in the perceived importance of the study
  - loss of clinical autonomy
  - incompatibility of protocol with normal clinical practice
  - problems in complying with the protocol
  - problems with the consent procedure.
- **Patients**
  - additional demands of:
    - extra procedures
    - time commitment
    - travel
  - patient preferences
  - worry about acknowledged uncertainty
  - concerns about information and consent.

Conduct

Recruitment of participants

No prospective survey of problems which occur in the conduct of randomised trials has been identified. Perhaps 20% of planned RCTs never start, mainly because of a lack of funding or logistical problems.[10] Of those that do, more than 50% have difficulty with recruitment[11] which can lead to abandonment or reduced size and hence loss of statistical power. Proposed solutions to poor recruitment include piloting, the use of multiple strategies to screen at least twice the planned sample size, contingency plans if recruitment is slow, and the use of recruitment coordinators. None of these has been rigorously evaluated. For multicentre randomised trials, there is little evidence to support excluding so called non-expert centres.[12] Staggered entry of centres may reduce the effects of recruitment fatigue.[13]

Concealment of allocation

Failure to ensure and to audit adequate concealment of random allocation to groups has been associated with bias (Box 8.4).[8]

Box 8.4 Poor concealment of allocation at randomisation is associated with bias

Schulz *et al.*[8] evaluated the methodological quality of 250 randomised controlled trials from 33 meta-analyses and then analysed the associations between those assessments and estimated treatment effects. Randomised trials in which concealment of allocation was either inadequate or unclear yielded larger estimates of treatment effects than those in which allocation was considered to have been adequately concealed (for example, central randomisation, numbered or coded bottles or containers, or serially numbered opaque sealed envelopes). Odds ratios were exaggerated by 41% in inadequately concealed studies and by 30% for unclearly concealed studies.

Compliance

Inadequate compliance with the study protocol can lead to false-negative or false-positive results.[14,15] Unfortunately, methods to improve the compliance with RCT protocols have not been rigorously evaluated. Some assessment of the compliance both of clinicians and participants should be made but it can be difficult to measure.[14]

Blinding

Placebos are widely used to blind the patients and health care professionals but there is evidence from drug trials that participants are frequently unblinded by side effects.[16] This raises the potential for bias, especially with subjective outcomes, but there have been few well-documented cases. Establishing that blinding has been successful is reassuring but there is no consensus on what to do if the blinding has failed. Blinded outcome assessment is particularly important, as in many situations it is the only blinding which is possible. Unblinded outcome assessment is demonstrably associated with bias in some situations.[17,18]

Follow-up

Follow-up should be attempted for all patients randomised to minimise attrition bias but many surveys of RCTs have shown that this does not occur (up to 70% of randomised trials in some areas excluded more than 15% of patients after randomisation). Monitoring can identify patients who have missed follow-up so that they can be contacted. Outcomes should be kept to a minimum.

Quality control

Quality control is clearly important[19] but too much may make randomised trials prohibitively expensive and hinder recruitment. However, there is little evidence to support or refute intensive quality control measures. One RCT has compared double versus single data entry and, although there were fewer errors with double entry, most of these were unlikely to alter the results significantly.[20]

RCTs need a good organisational and administrative base but there has been little research evaluating the optimal structure. The precise roles of steering committees and data monitoring committees have been poorly evaluated. The latter improve the conduct of interim analyses: one non-random comparison showed that open reporting of interim results reduced recruitment and increased the number of RCTs stopped inappropriately compared to those with no open reporting.[21]

There is particular concern about bias in the design, conduct, and analysis of commercially sponsored trials, and there is some (largely anecdotal) evidence to support this.[22] It may therefore be in the interests of sponsors, researchers, funders, providers, and consumers for these studies to have independent steering and data monitoring committees, and even independent data management and analysis.

Analysis

Intention-to-treat analysis

Intention-to-treat analysis is the method of choice to provide an unbiased estimate of treatment effects unless there are large and uneven losses to follow-up, when attrition bias may still operate. The confidence intervals of a treatment effect may differ sufficiently to alter the interpretation of the results when only analysis by protocol completion is reported.[3] Consideration should be given to reporting both analyses with the supporting data provided.

Multiple testing and subgroup analysis

Regulatory bodies have dealt with the problem of multiple significance testing by imposing a requirement to identify in a study protocol a primary outcome, supplemented by predetermined secondary outcomes. A clear statistical plan is another essential for regulatory bodies and this should also be made compulsory before approval to proceed with a randomised trial is given by funders or ethics committees. Any subgroup analyses that are proposed as hypothesis testing should be specified in the protocol and the study must be of sufficient size to detect such an interaction. All other subgroup analyses should be considered as hypothesis generating.

Reporting

At least 25 surveys have demonstrated that many RCTs are poorly reported, making it difficult to assess the quality of their methods. The recent development of the CONSORT guidelines should improve reporting,[23] although they will need to be updated from time to time. Evidence from cardiovascular medicine has shown that physicians are more likely to view treatments as effective if presented with relative rather than absolute risks, although the latter are more clinically relevant.[24,25] Both measures should therefore be presented.

There is some evidence that the conclusions of a report are frequently not supported by the data presented, particularly for commercially sponsored studies.[26] Despite worries over the potential for bias in commercially sponsored randomised trials, there are few studies describing the adequacy of reporting of commercial involvement. Results should ideally be presented in the context of a systematic review of previous similar RCTs, but this has rarely been done.

About 10% of completed RCTs remain unpublished whilst many others are only published in conference proceedings, particularly if the studies are small and have shown small, non-significant treatment effects.[27,28] Such publication bias is a major problem, especially for those trying to summarise all the research evidence in systematic reviews. The only adequate solution is likely to be prospective registration of all randomised trials. Paradoxically, multiple publication of the same study is also a problem for those showing significant results.[29] Journal editors should insist that all previous publications of a randomised trial are referenced in the report.

Costs

Treatment costs
Economic outcomes are often as relevant as clinical outcomes in health technology assessment. Although many authors have

advocated cost-effectiveness analysis, few RCTs have reported an economic evaluation. This may be due both to the difficulties in doing so (additional data collection, limited access to economic expertise) and to the lack of generalisability from one health care context to another. Although some components of an economic analysis are subject to uncertainty, results are often interpreted as if they are known with certainty. Therefore, statistical tests and confidence intervals should be used. Sample size calculations should take the economically important effect size into account (Box 8.5).[30]

Box 8.5 Prior economic modelling can increase the efficiency of randomised trials

Technologies which cannot be more cost-effective than other options, no matter how clinically effective they are, should not be subjected to randomised trials. Torgerson *et al.*[31] advocated economic modelling of the potential cost-effectiveness of health care interventions to prevent hip fractures from osteoporosis. A single annual vitamin D injection may be the most cost-effective method of preventing hip fractures amongst the various strategies which have been proposed. Daily calcium and vitamin D is the only other treatment that is likely to merit evaluation in a randomised trial.

Research costs

Most of the literature on research costs in RCTs is from North America. Several studies have compared the cost-effectiveness of different recruitment strategies, but no consistent finding has emerged. The costs of carrying out a diagnostic or therapeutic intervention may deter recruitment. In North America, the costs of extra tests may fall upon the patient or the purchaser. In the United Kingdom, the cost to the National Health Service of caring for patients in randomised trials may be perceived as an unaffordable new service, delaying or preventing recruitment in some participating centres.

Recommendations

- Researchers should:
  - undertake a systematic review of existing evidence before planning a new randomised trial;

- choose clinical, final outcomes rather than intermediate outcome measures;
- always provide detailed sample size calculations and a statistical plan;
- if the costs of the interventions differ, possibly calculate the minimum effect size compatible with the more expensive treatment being cost-effective;
- plan recruitment strategies and contingencies in detail;
- ensure adequate concealment of randomisation in order to avoid selection bias;
- create simple research protocols with straightforward data collection.
- Funders and ethics committees should:
  - ensure that dedicated research staff are available to support the clinical staff in conducting the study;
  - in phase III trials, including commercially sponsored trials, appoint independent steering and data monitoring committees;
  - create a system of prospective registration of all randomised trials.
- Journal editors should:
  - ensure that guidelines such as CONSORT are followed when randomised trials are reported;
  - insist that any previous publication of a randomised trial is referenced in the definitive report of the study.

References

1. Yusuf S, Held P, Teo KK, Toretsky ER. Selection of patients for randomized controlled trials: implications of wide or narrow eligibility criteria. *Statist Med* 1990;**9**:73–86.
2. Fleming TR, DeMets DL. Surrogate end points in clinical trials: are we being misled? *Ann Intern Med* 1996;**125**:605–13.
3. Henry D, Robertson J, Gillespie W, O'Connell D, Cumming R. *Meta-analysis of interventions for prevention and treatment of post-menopausal osteoporosis and fracture.* Report to the Australian Institute of Health and Welfare July 1995.
4. Gillespie WJ, Henry DA, O'Connell DL, Lau EM, Robertson J. Vitamin D analogues in the prevention of fractures. In: *Musculoskeletal Injuries Module of The Cochrane Database of Systematic Reviews*, Vol.3, 1996.
5. Klein KB. Controlled treatment trials in the irritable bowel syndrome: a critique. *Gastroenterology* 1988;**95**:232–41.
6. Wilensky AJ. Protocol design. *Epilepsy Res* 1993;**10**(Suppl.):107–13.
7. Silagy CA, Jewell D. Review of 39 years of randomised controlled trials in the British Journal of General Practice. *Br J Gen Pract* 1994;**44**:359–63.
8. Schulz KF, Chalmers I, Hayes RJ, Altman DG. Empirical evidence of bias. Dimensions of methodological quality associated with estimates of treatment effects in controlled trials. *J Am Med Assoc* 1995;**273**:408–12.

9. Fayers PM, Machin D. Sample size: how many patients are necessary? [editorial]. *Br J Cancer* 1995;**72**:1–9.
10. Easterbrook PJ, Matthews DR. Fate of research studies. *J Roy Soc Med* 1992; **85**:71–6.
11. Charlson ME, Horwitz RI. Applying results of randomised trials to clinical practice: impact of losses before randomisation. *Br Med J* 1984;**289**:1281–4.
12. Hjorth M, Holmberg E, Rodjer S, Taube A, Westin J. Patient accrual and quality of participation in a multicentre study on myeloma: a comparison between major and minor participating centres. *Br J Haematol* 1995;**91**:109–15.
13. Winkler G, Levin EA, Whalen EY, Larus J. Overcoming "trial fatigue": a strategy for optimizing patient accrual speed and resource utilization. *Drug Inform J* 1996;**30**:35–40.
14. Melnikow J, Kiefe C. Patient compliance and medical research: issues in methodology. *J Gen Intern Med* 1994;**9**:96–105.
15. Vander Stichele R. Measurement of patient compliance and the interpretation of randomised clinical trials. *Eur J Clin Pharmacol* 1991;**41**:27–35.
16. Fisher S, Greenberg RP. How sound is the double-blind design for evaluating psychotropic drugs? *J Nervous Mental Dis* 1993;**181**:345–50.
17. Carroll KM, Rounsaville BJ, Nich C. Blind man's bluff: effectiveness and significance of psychotherapy and pharmacotherapy blinding procedures in a clinical trial. *J Consulting Clin Psychol* 1994;**62**:276–80.
18. Noseworthy JH, Ebers GC, Vandervoort MK, Farquhar RE, Yetisir E, Roberts R. The impact of blinding on the results of a randomized, placebo-controlled multiple sclerosis clinical trial. *Neurology* 1994;**44**:16–20.
19. Poy E. Objectives of QC systems and QA function in clinical research. *Quality Assurance* 1993;**2**:326–31.
20. Reynolds-Haertle RA, McBride R. Single vs double data entry in CAST. *Controlled Clin Trials* 1992;**13**:487–94.
21. Green SJ, Fleming TR, O'Fallon JR. Policies for study monitoring and interim reporting of results. *J Clin Oncol* 1987;**5**:1477–84.
22. Julian D. Trials and tribulations. *Cardiovasc Res* 1994;**28**:598–603.
23. Andrew E, Anis A, Chalmers T *et al.* A proposal for structured reporting of randomized controlled trials. *J Am Med Assoc* 1994;**272**:1926–31.
24. Bucher HC, Weinbacher M, Gyr K. Influence of method of reporting study results on decision of physicians to prescribe drugs to lower cholesterol concentration. *Br Med J* 1994;**309**:761–4.
25. Naylor CD, Chen E, Strauss B. Measured enthusiasm: does the method of reporting trial results alter perceptions of therapeutic effectiveness? *Ann Intern Med* 1992;**117**:916–21.
26. Rochon PA, Gurwitz JH, Simms RW *et al.* A study of manufacturer-supported trials of nonsteroidal anti-inflammatory drugs in the treatment of arthritis. *Arch Intern Med* 1994;**154**:157–63.
27. Dickersin K, Min YI. Publication bias: the problem that won't go away. *Ann N Y Acad Sci* 1993;**703**:135–48.
28. Scherer RW, Dickersin K, Langenberg P. Full publication of results initially presented in abstracts. A meta-analysis. *J Am Med Assoc* 1994;**272**:158–62, 1410.
29. Keirse MJ, Van Hoven M. Reanalysis of a multireported trial on home uterine activity monitoring. *Birth* 1993;**20**:117–22.
30. Torgerson DJ, Ryan M, Ratcliffe J. Economics in sample size determination for clinical trials. *Qu J Med* 1995;**88**:517–21.
31. Torgerson DJ, Donaldson C, Reid DM. Using economics to prioritise research: a case study of randomised trials for the prevention of hip fractures due to osteoporosis. *J Health Serv Res Policy* 1996;**1**:141–6.

9 Ethics of randomised trials

SARAH JL EDWARDS, RICHARD J LILFORD,
DAVID A BRAUNHOLTZ,
JENNIFER C JACKSON, JENNY HEWISON
AND JIM THORNTON

We have conducted a systematic review of the literature which addresses the ethics of conducting RCTs. The literature was of two types, moral arguments and empirical studies. The main moral arguments deal with three issues:

- "uncertainty" as a basic justification for trials;
- the invitation to participate (consent); and
- interim analysis and deciding when to stop a trial.

The empirical literature aims to inform moral arguments by, for example, studying the effects of RCTs on those offered entry. In this chapter, we try to distinguish clearly between the findings of the review and our comments about the findings.

Nature of the evidence

Articles were classified according to whether or not they included empirical data. A total of 449 articles discussed the ethics of RCTs. An additional 169 contained empirical data. Here we deal with one or more of the following:

- the effects on anxiety, knowledge, and recruitment of different methods of inviting patients to participate in randomised trials (14 studies of which 11 used randomised designs);
- audit of whether people participating in randomised trials had understood the nature of their treatment allocation (24 studies);

- attitudes of patients, the public, and health care professionals (59 studies); and
- physical and psychological effects of randomised trials (14 and 3 studies respectively).

Our search also identified six reviews of empirical evidence on one or more of the above topics.[1-6]

Findings

Uncertainty as justification for randomised trials

The main reason given in the literature for using the RCT design is a scientific one: properly conducted RCTs produce valid data from which society benefits. Criticism of this as to the sole aim of medicine constitutes the most widely cited attack on RCTs and is based on the claim that the interests of participants are necessarily subjugated for the common good, that is participants pay the price for the benefit of future patients. The most widely cited counterargument is that patients are not asked to sacrifice themselves for the benefit of society if the treatments are an equal bet in prospect.[7]

In this context, "equipoise" has a more precise meaning than uncertainty.[7] "Uncertainty" is ambiguous in two respects. First, knowledge comes in degrees and therefore uncertainty includes many possibilities, a concept represented by a Bayesian prior probability distribution (Chapter 14). Second, when a known side effect of treatment must be traded-off against possible benefits, uncertainty may relate not only to the "prior" beliefs about the benefits but also to how they are valued.[7] Equipoise implies that expected gains are commensurate with side effects (perceived risks) of comparator treatments, that is the expected utilities of other treatments are the same and the participant does not lose out in prospect. It has been argued that, while equipoise has a precise meaning, the concept is elusive in practice since its measurement is inevitably imprecise.[8] However, it is our opinion that it provides a clear goal to aim at in contrast to the ambiguous term "uncertainty".

Further argument concerns the moral significance of different types of equipoise, collective and individual.[7,9] Freedman[9] has argued that equipoise among a group of relevant clinicians (collective equipoise) is necessary and sufficient to make a

99

randomised trial ethical, even if the individual clinician has a preference. Others[10] point out that patients may wish to know what their practitioner thinks or to make up their own mind on the basis of available evidence. Where trade-offs are concerned, equipoise depends on both prior beliefs and values, and it cannot therefore be determined outside the consulting room.[7,11] Equipoise is typically a property of the *patient*, rather than of the doctor, and equipoise among participating individuals is the ethical basis of randomised trials. The invitation to participate (informed consent procedure) is therefore critical (see below).

Recognition of the central role of equipoise as the moral basis of randomised trials has some radical implications.

- Small randomised trials are not necessarily unethical in their use of subjects, although they may offer poor value for money.[12]
- It is unethical to conduct placebo-controlled randomised trials in the face of a known advantageous treatment, which would otherwise be freely available,[13] or to repeat randomised trials simply to replicate positive findings.[14]
- The null hypothesis seems a poor rationale for statistical tests in circumstances where trade-offs occur. In these circumstances, RCT participants have prior expectations of benefits sufficient to compensate for expected costs. The most interesting hypothesis is therefore whether or not the data are compatible with the expectations of benefit. The null hypothesis is not the default position.

The invitation to participate

Informed consent is fundamental to the ethics of randomised trials. Numerous authors point out that, for informed consent to be valid, it must be competent, voluntary, not only technically but also in spirit, and all relevant information must be divulged. Since equipoise turns on personal values, its presence or absence may only be determined through detailed discussion. Some authors add that clinicians and researchers have a *potential* conflict of interests (between the individual and society) and, by eliciting the patient's own values, the risk of this becoming a real conflict is minimised. Many authors have argued that the goal of disclosing *all* relevant information is imperfectly realised in practice but we still have to decide what *ought* to be done. There are, nevertheless, many

Box 9.1 When consent cannot be obtained

The goal of full disclosure to an individual patient has to be compromised when the potential participant is not competent, for example because of unconsciousness or cognitive impairment. In these circumstances, a surrogate (relative or partner) is the best source of values since we may reasonably assume parity of interests and that the surrogate may have insight into what the patient would have wanted. Seeking consent from a surrogate means that the patient is not excluded from the opportunity to help others. However, in the absence of a surrogate or in an emergency, some have argued that randomisation should be avoided,[15] notwithstanding the large societal costs of doing so. Others, including the Medical Research Council,[16] and the Royal College of Physicians in the UK, and the Food and Drug Administration in the USA[17] have argued that, since normal practice must proceed on the basis of "assumed" preferences (that is, those of the "average" patient), randomisation may be ethical but only if the clinician is in equipoise with respect to his/her opinion of the patient's best interests and a proxy gives 'consent'. In some cases, it is possible to elicit consent in advance of a situation which may arise some time in the future. For example, a pregnant woman may give consent for scenarios that may arise in labour or the early neonatal period.

Box 9.2 Ethics of cluster randomised trials

Cluster trials involve randomisation of groups eg schools or hospitals. In some cases (type A), the intervention is also given at the group level eg flouridation of a water supply. Here, consent must be given for the group as a whole by a cluster 'guardian', such as a head teacher or hospital director, though it may be necessary for him/her to consult widely before deciding. In other cases (type B), randomisation is at the group level, but the intervention is administered to individuals – this is typically used for administrative convenience or to avoid the risk of contamination between one individual and another in educational interventions. Such trials are only ethical if they do not remove pre-existing choices.

situations where it could be argued that the *goal* of full disclosure to a participant should be relaxed, for example when consent is sought from a surrogate because a participant is not competent (Box 9.1) or is a member of a group in a cluster randomised trial (Chapter 11) (Box 9.2), or when disclosure of the treatment

---

Box 9.3 Consent and behavioural interventions

The goal of full disclosure may sometimes undermine the objective of a randomised trial, whether randomised at the level of individuals or clusters. When participants cannot be blinded, knowledge of the treatment comparison can introduce bias through differential changes in the behaviour or attitudes of the treatment groups.[18] This situation often occurs with educational interventions. Knowledge of the intervention amongst control subjects can lead them to seek the intervention outside the RCT, reducing the difference observed between groups or resulting in demoralisation, which is likely to depress outcomes for the controls and result in an exaggerated difference between groups.

A randomised consent design can be used in these situations,[19] although the design has been criticised from an ethical point of view. Randomisation is carried out prior to seeking consent, and consent is usually sought from those in the experimental arm. Controls might assent in ignorance of the detail.

---

comparison is likely to undermine the objective of the trial (Box 9.3).

A somewhat different situation arises when it is the fear of causing distress that inhibits free disclosure.[20] There may then be a trade-off between beneficence and autonomy. The obligation to respect autonomy is afforded greater importance in contemporary Western society where the essentially paternalistic Hippocratic tradition is not overriding. It has been cogently argued, however, that the option to relegate the decision remains a valid one; that is, the patient may ask the doctor to choose on his/her behalf.[21]

Effects of randomised trials on patients

For competent patients, it would be reassuring if comprehension, emotional well-being, and recruitment rates were positively correlated, implying harmony between individual and societal interests. However, empirical studies suggest that more information leads to better knowledge but lower consent rates (Chapter 6),[22] and greater, albeit transitory, anxiety.[23] However, the more background knowledge people have the less likely they are to be made anxious, irrespective of how consent is obtained.[24] Although many patients can answer questions about their randomised trial correctly, quantitative studies may overestimate how much patients have really understood. In a detailed qualitative study, many parents of critically ill babies did not know that they had consented to random allocation of treatment but thought that they would be receiving the new experimental therapy.[25]

Attitudes and the effects of randomised trials

We also sought empirical data on how patients, the public, and health care professionals view randomised trials. We found that slightly more people participate for personal gain than for altruistic reasons. This finding is consistent across studies and raises more questions since, given equipoise and available treatments, patients should neither gain nor lose by participating.[18] Do they not realise that they might end up as "controls"? Do they think that the "new and promising" treatment can only be accessed by participating in the study? The current data do not resolve this issue.

A substantial proportion of patients/members of the public thought that doctors would recruit people into randomised trials, even when equipoise was not present,[26] and some doctors "confessed" that they would be prepared to do so.[27] Some doctors reported not even telling patients that they were in a randomised trial, let alone giving them sufficient information: in one study 47% of doctors thought that their patients were not aware that they were to participate in a randomised trial despite having signed the consent form.[28] It is our view that using deception as a way of placing societal interests ahead of those of the individual patient is deplorable.

Further empirical data showed that randomised trials themselves may have a beneficial effect on patients' outcome both in terms of physical prognosis[5] and psychological experience.[29] What evidence there is suggests that RCTs are beneficial even when the experimental treatment was not superior to the control, provided that an effective treatment was already available.[18] The benefit appears contingent on the use of protocols which augment the quality of existing effective care.[18] This effect should not, however, be used as an argument to persuade an individual patient to accept randomisation; the Helsinki Declaration states that enhanced care should not be an *intended* consequence of participation. Nevertheless, as a society, we may gain reassurance from the evidence that well-conducted randomised trials tend to benefit participants.

Interim analysis

Issues arising from interim analysis have received much attention from the statistics community but little in the way of moral scrutiny. A moral issue arises because the results of RCTs, even interim ones, may dispel equipoise, thereby making future studies unethical. In order that beneficial treatments are detected as soon as possible and damaging ones are identified and rejected early, interim analysis is commonly used. Currently patients and practitioners are kept in ignorance,[30] with only a Data Monitoring Committee (DMC) being privy to preliminary results.

Data Monitoring Committees face a dilemma, since their role requires them to consider not only the interests of individual study participants but also society at large. If knowledge comes in degrees (as is conceptualised by a Bayesian framework – see Chapter 14), interim analysis may produce results that, while failing to reach prespecified levels of significance, nevertheless have the potential to destroy the equipoise that would otherwise exist. It is possible to model prospective benefit and harm to participants and future patients respectively, using interim analysis results and assumptions such as a "time horizon", before which the existing technology is not expected to be superseded.[31] However, this begs the question of how much the interests of society should be allowed to take precedence over those of potential participants. In the absence of a substantial body of ethical discussion on this point, we observe that DMCs have the seemingly impossible task of weighing the relative interests of trial and future patients, whether explicitly or otherwise.

We therefore support the view that interim analyses should be publicly available.[32] Disclosure need not necessarily thwart recruitment to the degree that may superficially seem inevitable. Doctor–patient pairs may move into equipoise, even as others move out. Accumulating data interact with different prior beliefs, and the resulting "posterior" beliefs interact with different individual utilities (values), such that recruitment and generalisability may actually be enhanced by the use of "feedback" randomised trials.[7] This is an empirical question.

Obligation of the doctor vs the policy-maker

In some conditions, it may still be ethical to start or continue randomisation even after effectiveness has been established, for example if the effective treatment is not available outside the RCT.[8] In this case, the individual doctor, who is bound by the Hippocratic Oath, is clearly acting in the patient's best interests by offering participation since the patient has some chance, rather than none, of getting the most effective therapy. From a societal perspective, this may also be justified if resources are scarce. However, in our opinion, it is unacceptable for a Data Monitoring Committee to withhold results simply to improve scientific precision, in the hope that this will change subsequent clinical practice. Public trust is fragile and we believe that it will disappear if doctors confuse their scientific and advocacy roles. Consent is an important safeguard in research for this very reason.

Recommendations

- Public confidence in RCTs can only be maintained if the practitioners can articulate clear, ethical justification for this method. This is only likely to be forthcoming if patients do not lose out in prospect, that is, if they are in personal equipoise or better.
- The empirical data show that most patients participate in randomised trials for non-altruistic reasons. This is possible when alternative treatments have equal expected utilities. Equipoise is therefore the proper basis of randomised trials of otherwise freely available treatments.
- Economy with the truth and suppression of values inherent in "uncertainty" (rather than equipoise) is unacceptable.
- The notion that societal interests should *not* take precedence over those of the individual is accepted by most authors, but gross violations of this standard have been documented.
- While practitioners are advocates for individual patients, governments, and other funders of health care must get the best buy for patients corporately. It may be ethical for funders to restrict expensive new treatments to randomised trials and license (or reimburse) only those technologies which have benefits that offset costs at a societal level.

105

References

1. King J. Informed consent: a review of the empirical evidence. *Inst Med Ethics Bull* 1986; December (Suppl. 3).
2. Meisel A, Roth L. Toward an informed discussion of informed consent: a review and critique of the empirical studies. *Arizona Law Rev* 1983;**25**:265–346.
3. Schain WF. Barriers to clinical trials 2: knowledge and attitudes of potential participants. *Cancer* 1994;**74**(Suppl. 9):2666–7.
4. Silva MD, Sorrell JM. Enhancing comprehension of information for informed consent: a review of empirical research. *IRB: Human Subjects Res* 1988;**10**:1–6.
5. Stiller CA. Centralized treatment, entry to trials and survival. *Br J Cancer* 1994;**70**:352–62.
6. Verheggen FWSM, van Wijmen Frans CB. Informed consent in clinical trials: review. *Health Policy* 1996;**36**:131–53.
7. Lilford RJ, Jackson JC. Equipoise and the ethics of the ethics of randomised controlled trials. *J Roy Soc Med* 1995;**88**:552–9.
8. Lockwood M, Anscombe GEM. Sins of omission? The non-treatment of controls in clinical trials. *Aristotelian Society* 1983;**57**(Suppl. LVII):207–22.
9. Freedman B. Equipoise and ethics of clinical research. *New Engl J Med* 1987; **317**:141–5.
10. Gehan EA, Freireich EJ. Non-randomized controls in cancer clinical trials. *New Engl J Med* 1974;**290**:198–203.
11. Llewellyn-Thomas HA, McGreal MJ, Theil EC, Fine S, Erlichman C. Patients' willingness to enter clinical trials: measuring the association with perceived benefit and preference for decision participation. *Social Sci Med* 1991;**32**: 35–42.
12. Edwards SJL, Lilford RJ, Braunholtz DA, Jackson JC. Why "underpowered" trials are not necessarily unethical. *Lancet* 1997;**350**:804–7.
13. Rothman KJ, Michels KB. The continuing unethical use of placebo controls. *New Engl J Med* 1994;**331**:394–8.
14. Senn SJ. Falsificationism and clinical trials. *Statist Med* 1991;**10**:1679–92.
15. Kapp MB. Proxy decision-making in Alzheimer disease research. *Alzheimer Dis Assoc* 1994;**8**:28–37.
16. Working Party on Research on the Mentally Incapacitated. *The ethical conduct of research on the mentally incapacitated.* London: Medical Research Council, 1991.
17. Symposium on Informed Consent. In case of emergency: no need for consent. *Hastings Center Report* 1997;**27**:7–12.
18. Edwards SJL, Lilford RJ, Braunholtz DA, Jackson JC, Hewison J, Thornton J. Ethical issues in the design and conduct of randomised controlled trials: a systematic review. *Health Technol Assess* (in press).
19. Zelen M. A new design for randomized clinical trials. *New Engl J Med* 1979; **300**:1242–5.
20. Tobias JS, Souhami RL. Fully informed consent can be needlessly cruel. *Br Med J* 1993;**307**:1199–201.
21. Dworkin G. *The theory and practice of autonomy.* Cambridge: Cambridge University Press, 1988.
22. Edwards SJL, Lilford RJ, Thornton J, Hewison J. Informed consent for clinical trials: in search of the best method. *Social Sci Med* (in press).
23. Simes RJ, Tattersall MHN, Coates AS, Raghaven D, Solomon HJ, Smartt H. Randomised comparison of procedures for obtaining informed consent in clinical trials of treatment of cancer *Br Med J* 1986;**293**:1065–8.
24. Aaronson NK, Visserpol E, Leenhouts GHMW *et al.* Telephone-based nursing intervention improves the effectiveness of the informed consent process in cancer clinical trials. *J Clin Oncol* 1996;**14**:984–96.

25. Snowdon C, Garcia J, Elbourne D. Making sense of randomisation: responses of parents of critically ill babies to random allocation of treatment in a clinical trial. *Social Sci Med* 1997;**45**:1337–55.
26. Cassileth BR, Lusk EJ, Miller DS, Hurtwitz S. Attitudes toward clinical trials among patients and the public. *J Am Med Assoc* 1982;**248**:968–70
27. Taylor KM, Kelner M. Interpreting physician participation in randomized clinical trials: the physician orientation profile. *J Health Social Behavior* 1987; **28**:389–400.
28. Taylor KM, Kelner M. Informed consent: the physicians' perspective. *Social Sci Med* 1987;**24**:135–43.
29. Mann AH. The psychological effect of a screening programme and clinical trial for hypertension on the participants. *Psycholog Med* 1977;**7**:431–8.
30. Freedman LS, Spiegelhalter DJ, Parmar MKB. The what, why and how of Bayesian clinical trials monitoring. *Statist Med* 1994;**11**:23–35.
31. Berry DA, Wolff MC, Sack D. Public health decision making: a sequential vaccine trial. *Bayesian Statistics* 1992;**4**:79–96.
32. Clayton D. Ethically optimised designs. *Br J Clin Pharmacol* 1982;**13**:469–480.

10 Implications of sociocultural contexts for ethics of randomised trials

RICHARD E ASHCROFT,
DAVID W CHADWICK,
STEPHEN RL CLARK, RICHARD HT EDWARDS,
LUCY J FRITH AND JANE L HUTTON

The most widely accepted source of evidence for the safety and effectiveness of treatments is the randomised controlled trial (RCT). The ethical status of the RCT is much debated, with particular attention being paid to the role of informed consent, the fairness of enrolling patients into the control arm of the trial, and the legitimacy of randomisation.[1] For the most part these concerns come from one of two sources. The first is philosophical: can these methodological requirements be ethically justified rationally? The second is more pragmatic: are randomised trials of this treatment at this time justified, either in cases where the treatment is already well understood, or where the need to use the treatment in all cases is urgent, or because the treatment is apparently harmful?[2]

The aim of this chapter is to consider the ethics of RCTs from a different perspective. Is there evidence of systematic objections to the use of randomised trials in particular areas of health care, where these objections are related to particular cultural or socioeconomic groups? For example, do members of some religious group object to randomisation *per se*, or is there evidence that RCTs are systematically unfair to some group, because they are recruited disproportionately? If such systematic objections exist, are there alternative methods for evaluating treatment which overcome these objections while retaining scientific validity, and can research ethics committees be made more sensitive to these issues?

Nature of the evidence

The study was a systematic review of two main kinds of literature: analytical studies of the ethics of randomised trials and empirical studies of evidence relating to cultural and socioeconomic attitudes to and experiences of such studies. We used a standard search algorithm to search MEDLINE, Socio-file and PsychLIT over the period 1990–1996; hand searching of the major medical and statistical journals; "explosion" of references in relevant literature; and library searching for books and articles of philosophical relevance. This generated in excess of 1000 articles, of which about 300 were used. There is no real literature that considers the ethics of RCTs specifically from a sociocultural perspective. There is a vast literature on their ethics in general and in particular areas of health care, much of which is repetitive, particularly about consent (over 300 articles, of which about 40 were usable).

Because of the indirect nature of much of our evidence, we have had to be quite cautious about the conclusions drawn. But while evidence is important in determining attitudes that should be respected, the feasibility of ethical proposals regarding consent, or in evaluating the consequences of some proposed action, ethics is also concerned with the validity and coherence of arguments, which has nothing to do with evidence. So we were able to construct arguments in this area with reasonable confidence, that can be considered as proposals for research and as hypotheses for future testing. Finally, if many of the ethical issues we identified philosophically currently lack an evidential basis, this is both a warning of problems that may arise, and a reassurance that our present ethical policies are currently reasonable (see Chapter 9).

Findings

We divided our findings into three main areas:

- methodological aspects of randomised trials from an ethical perspective;

- autonomy and informed consent in RCTs from a philosophical perspective; and
- cultural, economic and gender factors.

Methodological aspects of randomised trials from an ethical perspective

A number of ethical questions have been raised about the RCT. Is it fair to treat some patients differently from others? Is it fair to exclude some from the benefits of the new treatment, or to expose others to its harms? Is it fair not to treat some patients (those receiving placebos)? Is randomisation reasonable or even comprehensible? These questions fall into two basic types. The first type is methodological: given that it is unethical to enrol a patient into an experiment which cannot, in principle, do what is intended, does the RCT work? Because, if it does not, it is unethical. Some authors have attacked randomisation as unnecessary and ineffective, and some of them have gone on to conclude that even comparison between groups of current patients is unnecessary and unethical.[3] The second type is more directly ethical – even if the RCT were the most accurate source of evidence, it is substantively unethical.[4]

We reviewed the arguments about the scientific status of the RCT in order to settle the methodological question. Our conclusion, along with most scientists in this field, is that the RCT is the best available method for evaluating the effectiveness of most health care interventions.[5,6] Our main concern was whether there were any sociocultural objections to the randomised trial. It appeared that whatever objections there are to the method, these are not linked to any specific cultural groups. However, there are two issues which are important methodologically here: *if* some group were under- or overrepresented in RCTs, is this unfair and could anything be done to remedy that unfairness, and can anything be done to respect patient preferences about treatment? Both questions are important because, if there are some group-linked preferences about randomised trials, we need to find ways to accommodate these.

Preliminary answers to these questions suggest that there are occasions when some groups are overrepresented (in the US, especially the poor, who are often also from disadvantaged ethnic groups) or underrepresented (especially women, and in some cases, the poor).[7,8] Much can be done to make this selection fairer, but most arguments about the need to make samples socially representative for scientific reasons are false, and may introduce other biases.[9] Conversely, many existing studies may be not only unjust but also irrelevant because their findings cannot be generalised from the sample taken to the population where the treatment will be applied.[10] This argument from scientific validity is much more persuasive than the argument from social justice, and also more likely to satisfy social justice.

Autonomy and informed consent

No ethical concept is more widely known and debated than informed consent (or autonomous choice). This is reflected in the wealth of literature on this topic.[11] Its original role, in the Nuremberg code at least, was protective: to prevent people being experimented on without their knowledge, understanding, and agreement.[12] Since then, it has come to be the core of a whole rights-based approach to ethics in health care. We should distinguish between these two functions, the former procedural and the latter substantive.[13] In our review we were concerned about whether informed consent was actually a cultural universal: do all cultures accept it as an ethical obligation? Are there alternatives? For example, in the UK, we do not regard some people as competent or capable of consent – young children, or mentally incapacitated patients, for example. In other cultures, the groups excluded from competency may be different. Also, it is clear from the history of health care that informed consent, as an expression of the value of autonomy, has not always been accepted. We know that our own culture was, and others still are, more committed to paternalism as a good (for instance, in not revealing diagnoses of cancer to patients).[14,15] Finally, autonomy is a particular version of the conditions that are necessary for true consent; but it is also a highly individualistic concept, and not all cultures are individualistic.[16] This can be seen from the role played by the family or tribe in decision-making in many cultures (for instance, Mediterranean cultures, or the Inuit of Canada).[17]

Because of this variation, it was found helpful, following the philosopher John Rawls, to distinguish procedural understandings of consent from substantive understandings.[18] Procedural understandings concentrate on whether the parties to a decision

111

can regard the decision as having been made fairly, so that even if one party is unhappy about the outcome, they accept the process and agree to be bound by its outcome. The ethical content lies in the process. We take informed consent as a valid means for protecting patients, even if we have philosophical or other doubts about its status. The substantive understanding of informed consent – the autonomy theory – takes autonomy as a basic expression of human nature and its worth. Understood that way, it clearly does not command universal assent, and so cannot be universally ethically compelling – even if the substantive assumption is correct!

The main pragmatic worry about consent is the way the process can fail: either because consent is not sought, or because understanding can fail. There are some cases where obtaining consent is simply impossible, because the subject is unconscious, for example. Other tests of procedural fairness and patient protection can be used – minimal risk, substituted judgement, or best interests tests.[19] In a very few cases the research may require some deception but the requirements for prior agreement to take part in research and proper debriefing are very strict.[20] Arguments from inconvenience or difficulty in obtaining consent alone are insufficient.

The main ways that consent can fail are shown in Box 10.1. Whatever barriers there are on the patient's side, these may be reduced by a good quality consent process. The other side of this issue – paternalism – is promoted by assuming that these barriers to free consent cannot be overcome. There is no evidence at all for patients being largely irrational and so their decisions should be sought and respected.

Cultural, economic, and gender factors

Both the methodological aspects of randomised trials and the role of informed consent have been much studied, while the roles of culture, economics, and gender have not. The issues break down into: cultural attitudes to randomised trial design; cultural differences about consent; and justice.

There is some evidence that particular groups may object to experimentation on humans *per se* – there is certainly suspicion among many African-Americans resulting from the Tuskegee syphilis study.[23] This should be understood not as a cultural or philosophical objection to experimentation but as a failure of trust

Box 10.1 Main ways consent can fail in randomised trials

- *Paternalism* – assuming the consent is not in the patient's interest.
- *Overinterpretation* – if they agreed to that, they surely also would agree to this.
- *Language barriers* – not being familiar with the language used (either the language is not the patient's mother tongue, or the language is too technical).
- *Conceptual barriers* – not understanding the scientific concepts used (which can usually be simplified or clarified).
- *Social barriers* – not knowing that consent can be withheld, being in awe of medicine, being desperate, coercion by family. Also, in some health care systems, patients may not feel that they have any real choice, if they have the option of entering the study (and receiving free treatment) or not (and having to pay for treatment or go without).[21]
- *Psychological barriers* – risk aversion or risk attraction; gambler's fallacy (the luck of the draw will favour me); ignorance of one's own interests.[23]

in the system that conducts the experiments. In some instances this trust can be restored by the use of community consents.[24] There is also some evidence both that randomisation and the use of control groups may be regarded as unethical in some groups because these seem to rank scientific criteria above the obligation to do good to patients and to allow patients to control their own treatment. This has been an issue in some breast cancer and AIDS studies.[25,26] Apart from these examples, there is no available evidence for sociocultural objections to RCTs as such.

It has been thought that some cultures regard women as incompetent to give consent to treatment, but we could find no evidence for this in the literature, but we did find evidence for differential cultural attitudes to paternalism: some cultures expect more authoritative instruction from doctors than others.[27,28] Yet it is not clear that this is inconsistent with insisting on the consent test: paternalism rests on the idea that the doctor has expertise that I do not and is also better able to judge my best interests than I am, while consent rests not only on my right to make choices of treatment but also on my rights to refuse experimental treatment and to proper information about what decisions the doctor makes for me with my permission. Permission, even if implicit, is still essential. Nor is it clear that insisting on consent is actually harmful; the evidence that exists – albeit mainly from the UK or the USA – suggests that consent is generally beneficial. What does seem to be culturally variable is the role of the patient's family in decision-making. While we should insist that in the end the decision must be made by the patient, it is equally true that, where patients wish or need to consult with their family, they should be helped to do so, or arguably the quality of the consent is reduced.

Turning to justice, there is a consensus that patients should not be induced to participate in randomised trials, through payment of money or other benefits in kind, except perhaps as compensation for additional inconvenience incurred, but inequalities in wealth, health, and access to health care do occasion certain risks to some patients. If a person is poor and has no access to health care except through insurance or payment, then not only are they more likely to fall ill, they are also less likely to be able to pay, and so more likely to enter a randomised trial simply to gain access to treatment. In addition, they are more likely to live in the inner city and so near to teaching hospitals where research is a main activity. So they have a higher chance of being invited to participate in a RCT. Sometimes this unfair exclusion is reversed: a treatment may be evaluated in an affluent area because the baseline outcomes are likely to be better, so the poor get less access to novel therapies. While it is not at all clear how these unjust distributions of the risks and benefits of participation in an RCT can be remedied, it is certain that the problem needs consideration, especially in the international context.[29]

Recommendations

The main difficulty in making recommendations is a lack of evidence. Research is needed to discover underlying cultural and social attitudes to methodological elements of RCTs, particularly in the areas of justice in research planning, cultural attitudes to consent, and patient preferences and decision-making. Some broad recommendations are possible on the basis of existing evidence however.

- As in all areas of health care, the ethics of RCTs should place the patient's perspective and interests at the centre. This involves understanding and reflecting cultural and social parts of patient identity. This does not override the necessity of informed consent, so much as contribute to it.

- More attention needs to be focused on justice issues regarding individuals and communities. Some groups are overresearched, others underresearched, some unjustly excluded (intentionally or not), and others unjustly included.

- Consequently, research ethics committees should consider the cultural and religious groups in their locality, and become informed about the special issues that may arise regarding research involving members of these groups as individuals or populations.

- Research ethics committees should also ensure that research treats populations in their locality fairly – avoiding over-researching and other forms of social exploitation.

References

1. Ashcroft RE, Chadwick DW, Clark SRL, Edwards RHT, Frith L, Hutton JL. Implications of socio-cultural contexts for ethics of clinical trials. *Health Technol Assess* 1997;**1**(9):1–65.
2. Epstein S. Democratic science? AIDS activism and the contested construction of knowledge. *Socialist Rev* 1991;**21**:35–64.
3. Urbach P. The value of randomisation and control in clinical trials. *Statist Med* 1993;**12**:1421–41.
4. Lockwood M, Anscombe GEM. Sins of omission? The non-treatment of controls in clinical trials. *Aristotelian Society* 1983;**57**(Suppl. LVII):207–27.
5. Mike V. Philosophers assess randomised clinical trials: the need for dialogue. *Controlled Clin Trials* 1989;**10**:244–53.
6. Hutton JL. The ethics of randomised controlled trials: a matter of statistical belief? *Health Care Analysis* 1996;**4**:95–102.
7. McCarthy CR. Historical background of clinical trials involving women and minorities. *Academic Med* 1994;**69**:695–8.
8. Merton V. The exclusion of the pregnant, pregnable and once-pregnable people (a.k.a. women) from biomedical research. *Am J Law Med* 1993;**19**:369–451.
9. Senn SJ. A personal view of some controversies in allocating treatment to patients in clinical trials. *Statist Med* 1995;**14**:2661–74.
10. Ellenberg JH. Cohort studies: selection bias in observational and experimental studies. *Statist Med* 1994;**13**:557–67.
11. Faden RR, Beauchamp TL. *A history and theory of informed consent*. Oxford: Oxford University Press, 1986.
12. Annas GJ, Grodin MA (eds) *The Nazi doctors and the Nuremberg Code: human rights in human experimentation*. Oxford: Oxford University Press, 1992.
13. Engelhardt HT Jr. *The foundations of bioethics*. Oxford: Oxford University Press, 2nd edn, 1996.
14. Garnham JC. Some observations on informed consent in non-therapeutic research. *J Med Ethics* 1975;**1**:138–45.
15. Orona CJ, Koenig BA, Davis AJ. Cultural aspects of nondisclosure. *Cambridge Quart Healthcare Ethics* 1994;**3**:338–46.

16. Zion D. Can communities protect autonomy? Ethical dilemmas in HIV preventative drug trials. *Cambridge Quart Healthcare Ethics* 1995;**4**:516–23.
17. Verdun-Jones S, Weisstub DN. Consent to human experimentation in Quebec: the application of the civil law principle of personal inviolability to protect special populations. *Int J Law Psychiatry* 1995;**18**:163–82.
18. Rawls JA. *Theory of justice*. Oxford: Oxford University Press, 1971.
19. Karlawish JHT, Hall JB. The controversy over emergency research: a review of the issues and suggestions for a resolution. *Am J Respir Crit Care Med* 1996; **153**:499–506.
20. British Psychological Society. *Ethical principles for conducting research with human participants*. London: BPS, 1997.
21. Levinsky NG. Social, institutional and economic barriers to the exercise of patients' rights. *New Engl J Med* 1996;**334**:532–4.
22. Daugherty C, Ratain MJ, Grochowski E *et al.* Perceptions of cancer patients and their physicians involved in Phase I trials. *J Clin Oncol* 1995;**13**:1062–72.
23. Dula A. African-American suspicion of the healthcare system is justified: what do we do about it? *Cambridge Quart Healthcare Ethics* 1994;**3**:347–57.
24. Kymlicka W. *Liberalism, community and culture*. Oxford: Oxford University Press, 1989.
25. Kerns TA. *Ethical issues in HIV vaccine trials*. London: Macmillan, 1997.
26. Kotwall CA, Mahoney LJ, Myers RE, Decoste L. Reasons for non-entry in randomised clinical trials for breast cancer: a single institutional study. *J Surg Oncol* 1992;**50**:125–9.
27. Levine RJ. Informed consent: some challenges to the universal validity of the Western model. *Law Med Healthcare* 1991;**19**:207–13.
28. Ashcroft JJ, Leinster SJ, Slade PD. Breast cancer – patient choice of treatment: preliminary communication. *J Roy Soc Med* 1985;**78**:43–6.
29. Freeman HP. The impact of clinical trial protocols on patient care systems in a large city hospital: access for the socially disadvantaged. *Cancer* 1993;**72**: 2834–8.

11 Evaluation of health care interventions at area and organisation level

OBIOHA C UKOUMUNNE,
MARTIN C GULLIFORD, SUSAN CHINN,
JONATHAN AC STERNE, PETER GJ BURNEY
AND ALLAN DONNER

Health care interventions are often implemented at the level of organisation or geographical area rather than at the level of the individual patient or healthy subject. For example, screening programmes may be delivered to the residents of a particular area; health promotion interventions might be delivered to towns or schools; general practitioners deliver services to registered populations; hospital specialists deliver health care to clinic populations. Interventions at area or organisation level are delivered to clusters of individuals.

The evaluation of area or organisation-based interventions may require the allocation of clusters of individuals to different intervention groups (Box 11.1).[1,2] Evaluations of interventions in which clusters rather than individuals are allocated present a number of problems.[3] Often only a small number of organisational units of large size are available for study. The investigator needs to consider the most effective way of designing a study with a small number of study clusters. In cluster-level studies outcomes may be evaluated either at cluster level or at individual level (Box 11.2).[4] Cluster-level interventions are often aimed at modifying the outcomes of the individuals within clusters. It will then be important to recognise that outcomes for individuals within the

---

Box 11.1 Reasons for carrying out cluster-level evaluations

- Public health and health promotion programmes are generally implemented at an organisation rather than individual level, so cluster-level studies are more appropriate for assessing the effectiveness of such programmes.
- It may not be appropriate, or possible in practice, to randomise individuals to intervention groups since all individuals within a general practice or clinic may be treated in the same way.
- "Contamination" may sometimes be minimised through allocation of appropriate organisational clusters to intervention and control groups. For example, individuals in an intervention group might communicate a health promotion message to control individuals in the same cluster. This might be minimised by randomising whole towns to different interventions.
- Studies in which entire clusters are allocated to groups may sometimes be more cost-effective than individual level allocation, if locating and randomising individuals is relatively costly.

---

same organisation may tend to be more similar than for individuals in different organisational clusters (Box 11.3). Dependence between individuals in the same cluster has important implications for the design and analysis of organisation-based studies.[5] This chapter addresses these issues.

Nature of the evidence

We retrieved relevant literature using computer searches of MEDLINE, BIDS (Bath Information and Data Services) and ERIC (Education Resources Information Centre) databases and hand searches of relevant journals. The papers retrieved included theoretical statistical studies and studies which applied these methods. Much relevant work has been done on community intervention studies to prevent coronary heart disease. The content of the papers was reviewed, qualitative judgements were made concerning the validity of different approaches and the best evidence was synthesised into recommendations.[6]

Findings

We identified ten key considerations for evaluating cluster-level interventions.

Box 11.2 Comparison of levels of intervention and levels of evaluation[4]

		LEVEL OF INTERVENTION	
		Individual	Area or organisation
LEVEL OF EVALUATION	**Individual**	**Clinical study** e.g. Does treating multiple sclerosis patients with beta interferon reduce their morbidity from the condition?	**Area- or organisation-based evaluation** e.g. Does providing GPs with guidelines on diabetes management improve blood glucose control in their patients? Does providing a "baby-friendly" environment in hospital, increase mothers' success at breast feeding?
	Area or organisation		**Area- or organisation-based evaluation** e.g. Do smoking control policies increase the proportion of smoke free work places? Do fundholding general practices develop better practice facilities than non-fundholders?

Recognise the cluster as the unit of intervention or allocation

Health care evaluations often fail to recognise, or use correctly, the different levels of intervention which may be used for allocation and analysis.[7] Failure to distinguish individual-level from cluster-level intervention or analysis can result in studies which are inappropriately designed or which give incorrect results.[3]

119

Box 11.3 Three reasons for correlation of individual responses within area or organisational clusters

- Healthy subjects or patients may choose the social unit to which they belong. For example, individuals may select their doctors on the basis of characteristics such as age, gender or ethnic group. Individuals who choose the same social or organisational unit might be expected to have something in common.
- Cluster-level attributes may have a common influence over all individuals in that cluster thus making them more similar. For example, outcomes of surgery may vary systematically between surgeons, so that outcomes for patients treated by one surgeon tend to be more similar to each other than to those of another surgeon.
- Individuals may interact within the cluster, leading to similarities between individuals for some health-related outcomes. This might occur, for example, when individuals within a community respond to health promotion messages communicated through news media.

Justify the use of the cluster as the unit of intervention or allocation

For a fixed number of individuals, studies in which clusters are randomised are not as powerful as traditional RCTs in which individuals are randomised[5] (see below). The decision to allocate at organisation level should therefore be justified on theoretical, practical or economic grounds.

Randomise clusters wherever possible

Random allocation has not been used as often as it should have been in the evaluation of area or organisation level interventions. Randomisation should be used to ensure that the estimate of the effect of an intervention is not biased as a result of confounding with known or unknown variables. There are occasions when the investigator will not be able to control the assignment of clusters, for example when evaluating an existing service,[8] but because of the risk of bias, use of non-randomised designs should always be justified (Chapters 6 and 7).

Include a sufficient number of clusters

Evaluation of an intervention which is implemented in a single cluster will not usually give generalisable results. For example, a study evaluating a new way of organising care at one diabetic clinic would actually be an audit, from which generalisable observations may be difficult. A comparison between control and intervention clinics, with only one clinic per group would also be of little value, since the effect of the intervention is completely confounded with the underlying variation in response between the two clinics. Studies with only a few (less than four) clusters per group should generally be avoided as the sample size will be too small to allow a valid statistical analysis with an appreciable chance of detecting an intervention effect.[9] Studies with as few as six clusters per group have been used to demonstrate effects from cluster-based interventions,[10] but larger numbers of clusters will often be needed particularly when relevant intervention effects are small.[11]

Allow for clustering when estimating the required sample size

When evaluating cluster-level interventions by means of observations made at the individual level, standard sample size formulae will underestimate the total number of individuals required. Underestimation occurs because the standard formulae assume that the responses of individuals within clusters are independent (Box 11.3),[5,12–16] that is, variation *within clusters* is allowed for, but variation *between clusters* is not.

In order to allow for the correlation between subjects, sample sizes calculated by conventional formulae should be increased by a multiple known as the design effect or variance inflation factor.[5,12–16] Increasing the sample size by this method allows a cluster-level evaluation to have the same power to detect a given intervention effect as a study with individual allocation.

The design effect (*Deff*) is estimated from the average cluster size (n) and the intraclass correlation coefficient (ρ):

$$Deff = 1 + ((n-1)\ \rho)$$

The intraclass correlation coefficient is the proportion of the total variation of the outcome that is between clusters; it gauges the degree of similarity or correlation between subjects within the

121

same cluster. The larger the intraclass correlation coefficient, that is the more similar the subjects are within a cluster, the greater the size of the design effect and the larger the additional number of subjects required in a cluster-based evaluation to compensate for the loss in power.

An estimate of the intraclass correlation coefficient is needed when planning a study; if it is not available, plausible values must be estimated. One of our recommendations is that researchers should publish estimates of the intraclass correlation coefficient for key outcomes of interest, for different types of individuals, and for different levels of geographical and organisational clustering.[17] This will aid the planning of future organisation level interventions. Some examples of intraclass correlation coefficients are given in Table 11.1.

The number of clusters required for a study can be estimated by dividing the total number of individuals required by the average cluster size. When sampling of individuals within clusters is feasible, the power of the study may be increased either by increasing the number of individuals within clusters, or by increasing the number of clusters. Increasing the number of clusters will usually enhance the generalisability of the study and will give greater flexibility at the time of analysis.[11] However, the relative cost of increasing the number of clusters in the study, rather than the number of individuals within clusters, will also be an important consideration.

Consider the use of matching or stratification of clusters where appropriate

Stratification entails assigning clusters to strata classified according to cluster-level prognostic factors. Equal numbers of clusters are then allocated, ideally by randomisation, to each intervention group from within each stratum. Some stratification or matching will often be necessary in area or organisation level evaluations because simple randomisation will not usually give balanced intervention groups when a small number of clusters is randomised. Stratification is only useful when the stratifying factor is fairly strongly related to the outcome.

The simplest form of stratified design is the matched pairs design in which each stratum contains just two clusters.[18] We advise caution in the use of the matched pairs design for two reasons. First, the range of analytical methods appropriate for the matched

Table 11.1 Examples of intraclass correlation coefficients for design of area or organisation-based interventions

Cluster type	Variable	Source of data	Unit type	Average cluster size	Number of clusters	Intraclass correlation coefficient	Design effect
District	Proportion of deliveries by elective caesarean section	Health service indicators	Delivery	4997	110	0·016	80·9
Town	Proportion of current smokers	ref. 28	Men aged 40–59	322	24	0·026	9·3
Postcode sector	Serum cholesterol	ref. 29	Adults aged 16+	17	711	0·023	1·37
Household	Serum cholesterol	ref. 29	Adults aged 16+	1·57	6948	0·17	1·10
Hospital	Mortality after upper gastrointestinal haemorrhage	ref. 30	Patients aged 16+ with upper gastrointestinal haemorrhage	74·9	74	0·006	1·44
General practice	Asthma related quality of life	Unpublished data	Patients with asthma	61·1	42	0·0098	1·59

design is more limited than for studies which use unrestricted allocation or a stratified design with at least two clusters in each group-stratum combination.[19] Second, when the number of clusters is less than about 20, a matched analysis will have less statistical power than an unmatched analysis, unless there is a very strong association between the matching variable and the outcome variable.[20] If matching is felt to be essential at the design stage, it is worth considering the use of an unmatched cluster-level analysis.[21] Stratified designs in which there are four or more clusters per stratum do not suffer from the limitations of the paired design.

Consider different approaches to repeated assessments in prospective evaluations

Two basic sampling designs may be used for follow-up; the cohort design in which the same subjects from the study clusters are used at each measurement occasion, and the repeated cross-sectional design in which a fresh sample of subjects is drawn from the clusters at each measurement occasion.[22-24] The cohort design is more appropriate when the focus of the study is on the effect of the programme at the level of the subject. The repeated cross-sectional design is more appropriate when the focus of interest is a cluster-level index of health, such as disease prevalence, because the new subjects sampled at follow-up are more likely to be representative of the clusters at the later measurement occasions, particularly for studies with long follow-up. However, the cohort design is potentially more powerful than the repeated cross-sectional design because repeated observations on the same individuals tend to be correlated over time, reducing the variation of the estimated intervention effect.

Allow for clustering at the time of analysis

Standard statistical methods are not appropriate for the analysis of individual-level data from organisation-based evaluations, because they assume that the responses of different subjects are independent.[5] Standard methods may underestimate the standard error of the intervention effect resulting in confidence intervals that are too narrow and probability values that are too small.

Comparisons of outcomes between intervention groups can be made at the level of the cluster, applying standard statistical methods to the cluster means or proportions, or at the level of the individual, using formulae that have been adjusted to allow for the similarity between individuals. The choice of level of analysis is sometimes referred to as the "unit of analysis problem".[7]

Individual level analyses allow for the similarity between individuals within the same cluster by incorporating the design effect into conventional standard error formulae that are used for hypothesis testing and estimating confidence intervals.[2,25] For adjusted individual level analyses the intraclass correlation coefficient can be estimated from the study data in order to calculate the design effect. About 20–25 clusters are required to estimate the intraclass correlation coefficient with a reasonable level of precision. A cluster level analysis will often be preferable when there are fewer clusters than this.

Allow for confounding at both individual and cluster levels

When there is a need to adjust the estimate of intervention effect for individual or cluster-level prognostic variables, then regression methods which allow for similarity between individuals in the same cluster should be used. The method of Generalised Estimating Equations treats the dependence between individual observations as a nuisance parameter and provides estimates of standard errors which are corrected for clustering. Random effects models ("multilevel models") allow explicit modelling of the correlation between subjects with the inclusion of both individual-level and cluster-level characteristics.[26,27] Random effects models were originally developed for use with continuous outcome variables. Some packages also provide logistic, Poisson, and other models. At present the estimation procedures for these models are approximate and have been reported to produce biased estimates in some circumstances. Regression methods for clustered data require a fairly large number of clusters but may be used with clusters that vary in size.

Include estimates of intracluster correlation and components of variance in published reports

For reasons presented earlier, estimates of the intraclass correlation coefficient are required for sample size calculation and should be published, together with between- and within-cluster components of variance.

125

Recommendations

Investigators will need to consider the special circumstances of their own evaluation and use discretion in applying guidelines to specific circumstances. We emphasise that the conduct of cluster-based evaluations may present unusual difficulties. The issue of informed consent needs careful consideration (Chapter 9). Interventions and data management within clusters need careful definition and standardisation. The delivery of the intervention should usually be monitored through the collection of both qualitative and quantitative information which may help to interpret the outcome of the study. Non-specific effects of intervention (Hawthorne effects) may deserve consideration. The withdrawal of clusters from the study may have serious implications for the analysis, and this should be considered at the design stage where possible.

1. Recognise areas or organisational clusters as the units of intervention.
2. Justify allocation of entire clusters of individuals to groups.
3. Randomise clusters to intervention and control groups whenever possible, and justify the use of non-randomised designs.
4. Include a sufficient number of clusters. Studies in which there are less than four clusters per group are unlikely to yield conclusive results.
5. Multiply standard sample size formulae by the design effect in order to obtain the number of individuals required to give a study with the same power as one in which individuals are randomised. Estimates of the intraclass correlation coefficient should be obtained from earlier studies.
6. Consider stratification of clusters in order to reduce error in randomised studies and bias in non-randomised studies. Some stratification should usually be used unless the number of clusters is quite large. Researchers should be aware of the limitations of the matched pairs design (that is, a design with only two clusters per stratum).
7. Choose between cohort and repeated cross-sectional sampling for studies that involve follow-up. The cohort design is more applicable to individual level outcomes, may give more precise results but is more susceptible to bias. The repeated cross-

sectional design is more appropriate when outcomes will be aggregated to cluster level, is usually less powerful but is less susceptible to bias.

8. Standard statistical methods, applied at the individual level, are not appropriate because individual values are correlated within clusters. Univariate analysis may be performed either using the cluster means or proportions as observations, or using individual level tests in which the standard error is adjusted for the design effect. Where there are fewer than about 10 clusters per group, a cluster-level analysis may be more appropriate.

9. When individual and cluster-level prognostic variables need to be allowed for, appropriate regression methods for clustered data should be used. Provided there are sufficient clusters, use of regression methods for clustered data may also provide a more flexible and efficient approach to univariate analysis.

10. Authors should publish estimates of components of variance and the intraclass correlation coefficient for the outcome of interest when reporting organisation level evaluations.

References

1. Koepsell TD, Wagner EH, Cheadle AC et al. Selected methodological issues in evaluating community-based health promotion and disease prevention programmes. *Ann Rev Public Health* 1992;**13**:31–57.
2. Donner A, Klar N. Cluster randomisation trials in epidemiology: theory and application. *J Statist Planning Inference* 1994;**42**:37–56.
3. Donner A, Brown KS, Brasher P. A methodological review of non-therapeutic intervention trials employing cluster randomisation, 1979–1989. *Int J Epidemiol* 1990;**19**:795–800.
4. McKinlay JB. More appropriate evaluation methods for community-level health interventions. *Evaluation Rev* 1996;**20**:237–43.
5. Cornfield J. Randomisation by group: a formal analysis. *Am J Epidemiol* 1978;**108**:100–2.
6. Slavin RE. Best-evidence synthesis: an intelligent alternative to meta-analysis. *J Clin Epidemiol* 1995;**48**:9–18.
7. Whiting-O'Keefe QE, Henke C, Simborg DW. Choosing the correct unit of analysis in medical care experiments. *Med Care* 1984;**22**:1101–14.
8. Black N. Why we need observational studies to evaluate the effectiveness of health care. *Br Med J* 1996;**312**:1215–18.
9. Salonen JT, Kottke TE, Jacobs DR Jr, Hannan PJ. Analysis of community based cardiovascular disease prevention studies – evaluation issues in the North Karelia Project and the Minnesota Heart Health Programme. *Int J Epidemiol* 1986;**15**:176–82.
10. Grossdkurth H, Mosha F, Todd J et al. Improved treatment of sexually transmitted diseases on HIV infection in rural Tanzania: randomised controlled trial. *Lancet* 1995;**346**:530–6.

11. Thompson SG, Pyke SDM, Hardy RJ. The design and analysis of paired cluster randomised trials: an application of meta-analysis techniques. *Statist Med* 1997;**16**:2063–79.
12. Donner A, Birkett N, Buck C. Randomisation by cluster. Sample size requirements and analysis. *Am J Epidemiol* 1981;**114**:906–14.
13. Donner A. Sample size requirements for cluster randomisation designs. *Statist Med* 1992;**11**:743–50.
14. Donner A. An empirical study of cluster randomisation. *Int J Epidemiol* 1982; **11**:283–6.
15. Hsieh FY. Sample size formulae for intervention studies with the cluster as unit of randomisation. *Statist Med* 1988;**7**:1195–201.
16. Shipley MJ, Smith PG, Dramaix M. Calculation of power for matched pair studies when randomisation is by group. *Int J Epidemiol* 1989;**18**:457–61.
17. Hannan PJ, Murray DM, Jacobs DR Jr, McGovern PG. Parameters to aid in the design and analysis of community trials: intraclass correlations from the Minnesota Heart Health Programme. *Epidemiology* 1994;**5**:88–95.
18. Freedman LS, Green SB, Byar DP. Assessing the gain in efficiency due to matching in a community intervention study. *Statist Med* 1990;**9**:943–52.
19. Klar N, Donner A. The merits of matching in community intervention trials: a cautionary tale. *Statist Med* 1997;**16**:1753–64.
20. Martin DC, Diehr P, Perrin EB, Koepsell TD. The effect of matching on the power of randomised community intervention studies. *Statist Med* 1993;**12**: 329–38.
21. Diehr P, Martin DC, Koepsell T, Cheadle A. Breaking the matches in a paired t-test for community interventions when the number of pairs is small. *Statist Med* 1995; **14**:1491–504.
22. Feldman HA, McKinlay SM. Cohort versus cross-sectional design in large field trials: precision, sample size and a unifying model. *Statist Med* 1994;**13**: 61–78.
23. Diehr P, Martin DC, Koepsell T, Cheadle A, Psaty BM, Wagner EH. Optimal survey design for community intervention evaluations: cohort or cross-sectional? *J Clin Epidemiol* 1995;**48**:1461–72.
24. Koepsell T, Martin DC, Diehr P *et al.* Data analysis and sample size issues in evaluations of community-based health promotion and disease prevention programmes: a mixed model analysis of variance approach. *J Clin Epidemiol* 1991;**44**:701–13.
25. Donner A, Klar N. Confidence interval construction for effect measures arising from cluster randomisation trials. *J Clin Epidemiol* 1993;**46**:123–31.
26. Rice N, Leyland A. Multi-level models: application to health data. *J Health Serv Res Policy* 1996;**1**:154–64.
27. Kreft IGG, de Leeuw J, van der Leeden R. Review of five multi-level analysis programmes: BMDP-5V, GENMOD, HLM, ML3, VARCL. *Am Statistician* 1994;**48**:324–35.
28. Shaper AG, Pocock SJ, Walker M, Cohen NM, Wale CJ, Thomson AG. British Regional Heart Study: cardiovascular risk factors in middle-aged men in 24 towns. *Br Med J* 1981;**283**:179–86.
29. Colhoun H, Prescott Clarke P. *The health survey for England.* London: HMSO, 1994.
30. Rockall TA, Logan RF, Devlin HB, Northfield TC. Variation in outcome after upper gastrointestinal haemorrhage. The National Audit of Acute Upper Gastrointestinal Haemorrhage. *Lancet* 1995;**346**:346–50.

12 Qualitative methods in health services research

ELIZABETH MURPHY AND
ROBERT DINGWALL

The growing interest in qualitative methods in health services research in the last 15 years raises some fundamental questions. Does such research really count as science? Do the outputs justify funding? What, if any, are the appropriate tasks for such research? How are its outputs to be judged? Can qualitative and quantitative research be combined?

These are not new questions. Although qualitative research is often presented as new, relatively untried and controversial, its history goes back several thousand years. For over 100 years, there have been self-conscious debates about its nature and value. Yet these questions remain unresolved. One problem which confronts investigators attracted by qualitative methods is the absence of a single authoritative answer. Conventionally trained researchers are likely to be frustrated by the lack of consensus.

Nature of the evidence

A systematic review of qualitative methods in the canonical sense is impracticable. Apart from the limitations of database coding, there is no agreement on a hierarchy of methods or even on the criteria for such a hierarchy. For example, focus groups have recently become popular with some researchers. Others think them useless because of the contaminating effects of group interaction. Some researchers evaluate methods by their ability to capture the subjective meaning of events to the people involved; others emphasise the difficulties of accessing other people's minds – we are not a telepathic species! This chapter takes a more traditional form, using professional judgement in an attempt to cover the major positions, to set them out fairly and to leave readers to judge what they find helpful and credible. In effect, it is a qualitative review of qualitative methods.

Findings

The contested nature of qualitative research reflects fundamental differences about the philosophy of science within the research community. All methods imply prior philosophical foundations (Box 12.1). However, a significant difference between qualitative

---

Box 12.1 What are qualitative methods?

- **Participant observation**
  The direct observation of naturally-occurring events and behaviour – in skilful hands and where feasible, this is the nearest to a gold standard in qualitative research
- **Conversation/video analysis**
  A refinement of observation using the ability to record and replay behaviour as a means of examining it in greater detail – best suited to fairly static settings where unobtrusive recording is possible and tends to trade breadth for depth
- **Text/discourse analysis**
  The examination of documents – papers, records, visual images, transcribed speech, etc. – as artefacts showing evidence of the history and culture of an institution
- **Interviews**
  More or less structured conversations about a range of topics negotiated between the interviewer and the informant, often taped and transcribed – best used cautiously as a supplement to observation to obtain data on less accessible events or to elicit particular types of account
- **Focus groups**
  A currently fashionable type of group interview whose validity remains controversial

---

and quantitative methods, is that, while the latter have established a working philosophical consensus, the former have not. This means that quantitative researchers can treat methodology as a technical matter. The best solution is one which most efficiently and effectively solves a specific problem. Once identified by experts, these "best solutions" can be disseminated to rank and file researchers as techniques which, mastered and faithfully implemented, ensure rigorous research. Qualitative research is different. Here, researchers' proposed solutions to methodological problems are inextricably linked to their philosophical assumptions. What counts as an appropriate solution from one position is fatally flawed from another.

The absence of consensus dictates caution in training qualitative researchers. The techniques of qualitative research appear simple, which, no doubt, at least partly explains its current popularity. It seems to demand only the everyday skills of watching, listening, and making sense of written material. However, novice researchers who ignore the foundational questions about methods will struggle to produce high quality work. It is the answers to these questions, rather than a set of technical rules, which discipline research practice.

Qualitative and quantitative methods

A fundamental argument within qualitative research is about whether or not reality exists "out there". Most quantitative researchers take the existence of external reality as read. There may be biases and distortions, which make it difficult to discover what is really going on, but there is something which we can study, however imperfectly. By contrast, some influential qualitative methodologists are profoundly sceptical about the existence of an independent reality. They reject the conventional notion of truth. What we take to be reality is either created or shaped by our minds rather than having an existence. Different minds perceive different truths and, in particular, different interest groups hold different versions of what is true in any situation. The fact that we achieve some consensus about what is true in a particular instance does not mean that we have discovered truth but that we have arrived at "socially and historically conditioned agreement".[1] For these constructivists, it is possible for multiple and even contradictory "truths" to exist side by side.[2]

The relativism of this position undermines the usefulness of research for practice.[3] If all that research can do is produce multiple, competing versions of the world, it is difficult to see why tax-payers' money should be spent on it. Novelists, poets, leader writers and armchair theorists can all produce versions of the world more cheaply.[4]

This is not to suggest that the search for truth is unproblematic. The idea that scientific observers can achieve unmediated objective contact with whatever they are observing is patently false. Descriptions of what is going on within a setting, whether by natural or social scientists or by lay people, are always shaped by the conceptual framework with which they approach the task. We can never approach an object or a setting *tabula rasa*. While, *what* the hospital manager and the hospital cleaner see going on is the same, *how* they see it is likely to be very different. In other words, there is one reality, but this can be represented from a range of perspectives. There is one truth, but there may be multiple versions of it. While reality may look different from different perspectives, competing versions cannot contradict one another and still be true. In our view, the responsibility of health services researchers who seek funding for their research is to pursue truth (whether through description or explanation) as rigorously as possible within the constraints which operate. We may never be able to know with absolute certainty that our conclusions are true, but this should not deflect us from the pursuit of truth as a "regulative ideal".[4]

Why use qualitative methods?

What are the grounds upon which health services researchers might choose to use qualitative rather than quantitative methods? How might qualitative and quantitative research methods be combined to produce results to inform policy-making and practice in the health service?

First, qualitative research is sometimes a useful precursor to quantitative research (Box 12.2). The randomised trial is conventionally taken as the gold standard in evaluative research. RCTs are most useful in establishing the effectiveness of certain kinds of fully specifiable and replicable interventions. The value of an RCT lies in the possibility of generalising beyond the setting in which the intervention has been tested. RCTs work well where the intervention is a drug-like entity which can be fully standardised. However, many important interventions do not conform to this model. For example, defining the intervention in a study of the effectiveness of counselling would be more problematic. It may be possible to standardise the setting, the length of the counselling

Box 12.2 Qualitative research as a precursor to quantitative research

Heritage and Sefi examined the ways which advice is given and received during the first visit by health visitors to first-time mothers, around 10 days after their babies' births.[16] They identified different patterns of advice-giving and observed that, within the consultation, some of these were more likely than others to elicit either passive or active resistance from mothers. Three quarters of all the advice-giving initiated by health visitors met with such resistance. As the authors acknowledged, it is not possible to extrapolate from mothers' verbal responses during the consultations to their subsequent decisions about whether to follow advice or not, but this study does suggest that much current advice-giving by health visitors may be ineffective.

It would be possible to develop an intervention study, drawing upon this work, to study the relationship between different kinds of advice-giving and the likelihood that mothers would follow the advice. In such a study, health visitors would be trained to use the patterns of advice-giving which Heritage and Sefi found to be associated with maternal acceptance rather than rejection. It would then be possible to compare the subsequent behaviour of mothers who were given advice in such ways and those who were not.

session, the qualifications of the counsellor and so on, but the counsellor's practice within the consultation is likely to be a critical factor in determining the outcome. A qualitative observational study of counselling sessions, carried out as a precursor to an RCT, would enable researchers to specify commensurable categories of practice, permitting the standardisation of the intervention required by experimental logic. The alternative is a premature operational definition of variables, meeting the conventions of the RCT but undermining the validity and, hence, the applicability of its findings.[5]

Secondly, qualitative research can be used to explain unanticipated or inconclusive findings from quantitative studies (Box 12.3). In health services research, an intervention which basic or clinical science suggests ought to be effective, may fail to produce the hypothesised benefit in its application. While randomised trials are effective in confirming that an intervention works, they are less useful for explaining unanticipated results. Qualitative methods

Box 12.3 Using qualitative research to explain unanticipated findings from quantitative research

The starting point for Bloor's observational study of the disposal decisions of Ear, Nose and Throat surgeons was the finding of marked geographical differences in the incidence of adeno-tonsillectomy.[17] Bloor analysed the decision rules which 11 ENT surgeons used to determine a child's treatment. For example, he found that specialists differed in the physical examinations which they carried out and the weight which they gave to examination findings as compared to history taking. Bloor's study shows how the systematic analysis of observational data can be used to identify the routine practices of health professionals, which have significant implications for their use of health service resources.

can uncover the contextual factors which modify the application of an intervention so that the hypothesised benefits do not materialise. They may also be used to explain apparently contradictory findings from similar studies. For example, findings about the effectiveness of therapeutic communities are inconclusive. Some evaluations suggest that these interventions are highly effective, while others find little benefit. Qualitative research can play an important role in showing what it is about one setting which works and what it is about another which does not. Such information is crucially important for people trying to implement the results of health services research.

A third role which is conventionally advanced for qualitative research is that of hypothesis generation (Box 12.4). The most significant contribution of qualitative research, it is argued, is in supplying hypotheses to be tested using quantitative methods. There is some truth in this, insofar as qualitative researchers' preference for a relatively open and unstructured research design allows theory to be generated from empirical data, with the result that the theory is more likely to fit and work.[6] This may indeed help to short-list hypotheses for testing in elaborate and expensive studies.

However, it is a mistake to assume that the usefulness of qualitative methods is restricted to the preliminary stages of research. Hypotheses and models generated in qualitative studies can be tested using either qualitative or quantitative methods. The

---

Box 12.4 Using qualitative research to generate hypotheses

Pope's paper is concerned with the day-to-day organisation and management of surgical waiting lists.[18] The author studied the management of waiting lists in one district general hospital, collecting data from a mixture of observation and interviewing. Pope identified a number of perspectives on waiting lists in the health services literature and tested two of these (that the waiting list is a form of queue and that the waiting list is more like a "mortlake" or pool of unmet need) empirically. In the case that she studied, she found that neither of these conceptualisations of waiting lists did justice to the ways in which lists were managed. She proposed that they were more appropriately likened to a "store", with admissions staff as the storekeepers. This model, she suggests, captures the activity and interaction of waiting-list management in ways which the previous concepts did not. As Pope herself acknowledges, this study is exploratory. Nevertheless it does suggest a number of hypotheses which might be refined and tested in subsequent qualitative or quantitative research. For example, it would be possible to take the model which Pope proposes and test its fit in other kinds of hospital with more or less complex managerial structures. It would also be possible to manipulate some of the factors which Pope has identified as contributing to the operation of a strict "first-come-first-served" mechanism in hospital admissions and measure the impact upon the service.

---

choice should be pragmatic rather than paradigmatic. Methods should be tailored to the hypothesis under study, rather than driven by prior commitments.

Judging the quality of qualitative research

How can the outputs from qualitative research be judged? There are no technical tricks that ensure the validity of findings. Validity does not lie in the slavish application of rules or algorithmic criteria. Various techniques, including member checking or respondent validation (asking the people studied to confirm the findings) and triangulation (using different methods to study the same issue) have been proposed,[7,8] but have been found to have fundamental shortcomings.[9–11]

The judgement of validity rests upon an assessment of the evidence that the researcher presents. It is particularly important that qualitative researchers give a clear exposition of their data collection process, allowing readers to exercise joint responsibility with them in judging the evidence upon which claims are based.[12]

Similarly, the analyst should describe the process by which the findings were derived from the data, clarifying the concepts and categories used in the research and demonstrating that the conclusions are justified.[13] Researchers should display enough data to permit an assessment of whether their analyses are indeed supported by the data. Readers will be more convinced of the validity of the analysis where alternative, plausible explanations have been considered.

Qualitative researchers emphasise the embeddedness of research data in the circumstances of their production. The analysis of data should therefore involve careful reflection upon the ways in which they have been shaped by the research process itself.[14,15] Such *reflexivity* will also take account of the researcher's own prior biases, recognising the role of values and prior assumptions in shaping any research account.

The credibility of reports will be strengthened where researchers demonstrate that they have engaged in a conscientious search for data which are inconsistent with their preliminary analyses. The search for *deviant* or *negative* cases allows researchers to refine their analyses until they can incorporate all available data.[14] Claims to validity are strengthened where researchers display negative cases in their reports, showing how these can be integrated into their analyses. It is the explicit search for falsifying evidence which strengthens the truth claims of qualitative research.

The validity of qualitative research is undermined where the perspective of any one group is presented as objective truth. *Fair dealing* should extend not only to the powerless within a setting, but also to the powerful.[13] Traditionally, qualitative research has been concerned with the underdog, but this risks failing to develop an evenhanded analysis. The credibility and usefulness of a research report will be enhanced where the analyst shows as much understanding of the powerful as of the powerless within a setting under study.

Recommendations

Qualitative methods have an important contribution to make to health services research. The decision about whether to employ qualitative or quantitative methods in tackling a particular research question should be made on instrumental and pragmatic grounds. The key question is not whether qualitative methods are better or worse than quantitative. Rather, we need to ask whether, given the resources available, qualitative or quantitative methods will provide the answers more effectively and efficiently. Likewise, the underlying criteria by which qualitative and quantitative research should be judged are identical. The first criterion relates to our degree of confidence that the research findings are true and the second concerns the usefulness of those findings in informing either policy or practice. The decision about whether qualitative or quantitative methods, or a combination of both, will produce the most trustworthy and useful findings is one which only can be answered in relation to a specific research problem in the light of the various considerations discussed in this chapter.

References

1. Smith J. The problem of criteria in judging interpretive inquiry. *Educ Eval Policy Anal* 1984;**6**:379–91.
2. Guba EG, Lincoln YS. *Fourth generation evaluation*. Newbury Park, CA: Sage, 1989.
3. Greene J. Qualitative evaluation and scientific citizenship. *Evaluation* 1996;**2**: 277–89.
4. Hammersley M. *What's wrong with ethnography?* London: Routledge, 1992.
5. Silverman D. *Interpreting qualitative data: methods for analysing text, talk and interaction.* London: Sage, 1993.
6. Glaser BG, Strauss AL. *The discovery of grounded theory: strategies for qualitative research.* New York: Aldine, 1967.
7. Sandelowski M. The problem of rigor in qualitative research. *Adv Nursing Sci* 1986;**8**:27–37.
8. Beck CT. Qualitative research: the evaluation of its credibility, fittingness and auditability. *West J Nursing Res* 1993;**15**:263–6.
9. Bloor MJ. Notes on member validation. In: Emerson RM, ed., *Contemporary field research: a collection of readings.* Boston: Little Brown, 1983.
10. Emerson RM, Pollner M. On members' responses to researchers' accounts. *Human Organiz* 1988;**47**:189–98.
11. Bloor MJ. Techniques of validation in qualitative research: a critical commentary. In: Miller G, Dingwall R, eds, *Context and method in qualitative research.* London: Sage, 1997.
12. Glaser BG, Strauss AL. The discovery of substantive theory: a basic strategy underlying qualitative research. *Am Behavioural Scientist* 1965;**8**:5–12.
13. Dingwall R. Don't mind him – he's from Barcelona: qualitative methods in health studies. In: Daly J, McDonald, I, Wilks E, eds, *Researching health care.* London: Tavistock/Routledge, 1992.
14. Silverman D. Telling convincing stories: a plea for cautious positivism in case studies. In: Glassner B, Moreno JD, eds, *The qualitative-quantitative distinction in the social sciences.* Dordrecht: Kluwer, 1989.

15. Hammersley M, Atkinson P. *Ethnography: principles in practice*. London: Routledge, 1995.
16. Heritage J, Sefi S. Dilemmas of advice: aspects of the delivery and reception of advice in interactions between health visitors and first time mothers. In: Drew P, Heritage J, eds, *Talk at work*. Cambridge: Cambridge University Press, 1992.
17. Bloor M. Bishop Berkeley and the adenotonsillectomy enigma: an exploration of variation in the social construction of medical disposals. *Sociology* 1976;**10**: 43–51.
18. Pope C. Trouble in store: some thoughts on the management of waiting lists. *Sociol Health Illness* 1991;**13**:193–212.

Part Three
Statistical methods

13 Statistical methods: good practice and identifying opportunities for innovation

DEBORAH ASHBY, SARAH J WHITE AND
PHILIP J BROWN

The systematic and efficient evaluation of technologies relies heavily on the use of appropriate methods and good statistical principles in the design, analysis, and interpretation of studies. Just as there is scope for developing and critically evaluating new health technologies, so there is scope for developing and critically evaluating statistical methods routinely used in health technology assessment. Statistical developments and innovations are often reported and discussed in a statistical forum, such as journals or meetings, and it can take a long time before new ideas become incorporated into standard practice. In this chapter, we review new developments in statistical methods, make recommendations about areas where new developments are ready to be put into practice, and highlight areas where there is currently inadequate research.

Nature of the evidence

To establish a baseline against which to judge what should be regarded as novel, we reviewed statistical guidelines currently in use in areas such as drug development. Guidelines for statistical practice tend to arise as a consequence of regulation, and so we acquired those developed for drug regulation. We also contacted pharmaceutical companies and other major research organisations. These guidelines formed the basis of our first review.

We then reviewed statistical developments for study designs, and statistical methods of analysis for studies that follow patients over time. We hand searched 10 relevant journals (*Statistics in Medicine, Journal of the Royal Statistical Society (Series A–D), Statistical Methods in Medical Research, Biometrics, Biometrika, Journal of the American Statistical Association, Controlled Clinical Trials*) for the years 1994 and 1995, classifying papers according to agreed criteria. This produced a database of 505 papers. To see how far the methods which we reviewed had been implemented in practice, we searched MEDLINE for the years 1993 to 1996 using keywords generated from the hand-searching phase.

One of the major problems was terminology, as words such as "longitudinal" and "survival" have both colloquial and more specialised meanings. Also, in medical publications, it is possible that sophisticated statistical methods are used, but given no prominence in abstracts or keywords, as the primary motivation for the publication is clinical.

Findings

Guidelines

Guidelines fall into three main categories; those developed for drug regulatory purposes, those developed by the pharmaceutical industry to ensure that working practices meet the regulatory guidelines, and those which are aimed at people involved in more general medical research.

Regulatory guidelines
Although pharmaceuticals are only one kind of health technology, they have a very important part to play. For historical reasons, the evaluation of new drugs has been more heavily regulated than any other technology, with formal procedures which need to be carried out in order to gain a product licence. As a result there has been more explicit discussion of acceptable practice, and it is here we found most in the way of written guidelines.

Historically, the licensing of new medicines has been regulated on a country-by-country basis. More recently there have been moves towards harmonisation at the European level, which has been followed by a move toward global harmonisation. The development of guidelines on various issues, including statistics, reflects these changes.

Most applied statistical work is currently carried out using what are known as "frequentist" (or "classical") methods, using confidence intervals and P-values to draw inferences from the data. By contrast, many statisticians argue for the use of "Bayesian" methods (Chapter 14) which provide a natural framework for accrual of evidence, with the potential to incorporate evidence external to the particular data set at hand.

A historical review of the regulatory guidelines reveals a growing recognition of statistical principles and an inferential framework. Guidelines from the USA,[1] published in 1988, made no explicit statement about an inferential framework, although references to "t-tests" and "95% confidence intervals" imply a frequentist approach. In general, the emphasis was on technique rather than principles. Guidelines drawn up by the Committee on Proprietary Medicinal Products[2] for European drug regulation explicitly acknowledged a predominantly frequentist viewpoint, whilst opening the door to other approaches. Two years later, guidelines produced by the International Conference on Harmonisation,[4] which were designed to allow consistency between US, European, and Japanese submissions, still made no explicit statement on inferential mode, but a detailed Annex on statistical methods again implied a frequentist framework.

Guidelines from the International Conference on Harmonisation on "Statistical Principles for Clinical Trials", soon to be released, emphasise principles as being more important than technique, and focus on minimising bias, and maximising precision and robustness. Inferential mode is explicitly acknowledged by the statement: "This guideline largely refers to the use of frequentist methods when discussing hypothesis testing and/or confidence intervals. However the use of Bayesian or other approaches may be considered when the reasons for their use are clear and when the resulting conclusions are sufficiently robust compared to the alternative assumptions." Guidelines for Safety Assessment of Marketed Medicines[5] outlined study designs and issues to be considered by company-sponsored postmarketing studies, and included little discussion on analysis.

Although most of the principles in these guidelines could apply to many study types, much of the detail applies to large-scale randomised trials. Issues particularly pertinent to RCTs, for example subgroup analysis, multicentre designs, and interim analysis, are discussed. They include very little on modelling strategies for more complex data such as survival or longitudinal data, although the need for explicit analysis plans, to avoid accusations of data-dredging, is emphasised.

Pharmaceutical industry guidelines

Researchers in the pharmaceutical industry have the responsibility to ensure that their work satisfies regulatory guidelines; this has often led to the development of standard operating procedures. Statisticians in the pharmaceutical industry have developed generic procedures[6] aimed at satisfying regulatory statistical guidelines, and individual pharmaceutical companies have also produced operating procedures which their employees must adhere to when involved in a clinical study. For some companies, operating procedures are detailed and represent a considerable investment in a very competitive market. For this reason, they are not in the public domain and cannot be reviewed in detail although, ironically, reviewing company material would probably give us the best overview of "standard practice". Without being able to review this material, we note the priority given to statistical procedures in the speedy evaluation of new medicines.

Academic research community

The academic research community is much less structured than the pharmaceutical industry and we have found relatively little formal statistical material. However, the main guardians of research quality are members of funding bodies, ethics committees, and editors of peer-refereed journals, and it is guidelines from these bodies that we have reviewed.

To ensure good quality statistics in publications, various journals issue statistical checklists which are used by authors or by referees reviewing manuscripts. Documents written by the UK Medical Research Council[7] and for members of Ethics Committees[3] have little detailed statistical content, referring to the role of statisticians instead. Journal guidelines, such as those for the *British Medical Journal*, are more detailed, but function more as checklists for design and analysis rather than as detailed prescriptions.

Review of study designs

The full evaluation of a new health technology requires many stages. To obtain a licence, a new pharmaceutical product must undergo extensive preclinical investigation in patients, including toxicity testing, and then be evaluated in short-term studies in patients and longer term RCTs to establish efficacy and safety. Even after a product licence is granted, postmarketing studies may be needed to investigate rare adverse events, or problems that only occur in long-term use. For non-pharmaceutical innovations, analogous investigations may be required, and the evaluation may be tied up in a complex way with changing or varying clinical skills and aspects of the delivery of health care (Chapter 20). In statistical language, there can be strong confounding.

Classifying papers was not a straightforward task, as statistical methods tend to be transferable; for example, many papers relevant to randomised trials may also be relevant to non-randomised studies. Table 13.1 shows the distribution of 378 papers which

Table 13.1   Distribution of papers by study design (n = 378)

Study design	No. of papers*
Preclinical trials	45
Randomised trials	275
Screening studies	25
Meta-analytic studies	15
Audit studies	5
Safety studies	6
Non-randomised studies	44

* The categories are not mutually exclusive, and therefore do not sum to 378.

could be regarded as being most appropriate for one or more study designs using our classification.

Preclinical studies do not fall into the arena of HTA, although they are important building blocks towards it, with their own specialised methods. Randomised and non-randomised trials, and meta-analysis can be used at various stages of research. In the area of randomised studies, there is work on cross-over trials, experimental design, multicentre trials, and equivalence trials. Meta-analysis is addressed in Chapter 16. Current work on screening includes the use of RCTs and methods for investigating potential biases, as well as mathematical modelling approaches to understand the complex issues involved in evaluating screening programmes.[8,9]

Explicit areas least frequently addressed are the evaluation of safety,[10,11] such as postmarketing studies, and audit. These areas are also considered only briefly by existing guidelines. The lack of material in these areas is disappointing because they are directly relevant to HTA.

Review of methods of analysis

The analysis of studies that follow patients over time fall into four main categories (Box 13.1). Studies of chronic diseases often require sequential measures of outcome, collected for example on a weekly basis, to characterise the true impact of different health technologies; measurements collected at several points in time are called longitudinal data. Studies of fatal diseases, or the occurrence of some other event of interest, such as an acute myocardial infarction, typically measure time to death or to the event; these are called survival data. Statistical methods for both of these topics are being studied (Table 13.2).

The statistical literature on longitudinal data is varied, with work on continuous and binary outcomes, and modelling of missing data.[16] In the health care literature 18 methodological papers were identified. Of all the papers mentioning longitudinal studies, 14% were in the field of psychiatry, 6% in AIDS/HIV, 5% in cancer, 4% in diabetes, with the rest spread over other clinical areas. Statistical literature on survival data consists largely of work on proportional hazards models and issues to do with study design. In the health care literature only eight methodological papers were found. Of all the papers mentioning survival, 32% were in the field of cancer, and 10% in heart disease, with the rest spread among a variety of clinical areas. The broad picture is that techniques for survival analysis have found their way into medical research, whereas techniques for longitudinal data have not yet "jumped" from the statistical to the medical research community on a large scale.

Recommendations

Our primary purpose in reviewing guidelines was to establish a baseline against which to judge what is new. We found that most guidelines stressed principles rather than details, raising the question of whether guidelines for statistical methods in HTA might be desirable. We found that, in contrast to drug development

Box 13.1 Examples of types of data used for studying patients over time

The occurrence of a specified event, such as death or the detection of metastases in patients with cancer of the colon,[12] is the focus of many studies and, particularly, RCTs of cancer treatments. *Survival data* measure the time between entry to a study and exit from it for each patient recruited. A patient can leave a study for a variety of reasons other than experiencing the event of interest, for example withdrawal or migration. These latter reasons are collectively called "censoring", the patient ceases to contribute survival time to the study, but the time to the most recent follow-up is included in the analysis.

Longitudinal data occur when an outcome of interest is measured on more than one occasion. An example is the measurement of CD4 counts at successive clinic visits in patients with HIV.[13] Longitudinal measures of quality of life are becoming increasingly important, and can be combined with survival data to evaluate the trade-off between quantity and quality of life in fatal diseases (Chapter 15).

More than one measurement is sometimes obtained for a patient for reasons other than follow-up over time. In this review we have called these *repeated measures data*. (The term repeated measures is sometimes used interchangeably with the term longitudinal data but we made a distinction between these types of data for the review.) For example, independent opinions may be sought from orthodontists on the need for extraction of children's teeth.[14]

A *time series* is a sequence of measurements over time, such as the number of new HIV notifications on a monthly basis.[15] When the primary interest is the analysis of an individual (long) series, time series are the most appropriate method. Analysis centres on identifying underlying trends and periodicity, for example seasonal effects, in the data, often with a view to prediction for the future. When there are (often quite short series) on many individuals, methods developed for longitudinal data (see above) are likely to be more appropriate. In both cases, the statistically important feature is the correlation between observations within a series, which must be appropriately modelled if correct conclusions are to be drawn.

where statistical thinking has matured to a stage where it can be encompassed in guidelines, the wider field of HTA is more embryonic. Statistical development, therefore, needs to take place alongside practical and other methodological developments in HTA.

Much statistical work is being carried out in the context of preclinical and long-term RCTs. By contrast, there is an extreme

Table 13.2   Statistical framework of papers that follow patients over time

Data structure	Statistical framework	No. of papers
Survival data	Frequentist	104
	Bayesian	3
	Both	1
Longitudinal data	Frequentist	43
	Bayesian	3
	Both	2
Repeated measures	Frequentist	12
	Bayesian	0
	Both	1
Time series	Frequentist	6

paucity of papers on safety assessment and audit, topics which contribute to the evaluation of technologies in everyday use. The development of statistical methods for studies of the safety of drugs and other technologies are a priority, and the development of statistical methods for audit is necessary.

Survival data are fundamental to the study of fatal disease and longitudinal data are fundamental to the study of chronic diseases. Methods for the analysis of survival data are relatively well developed and applied, but methods for analysing longitudinal data are still being developed and have yet to be widely implemented. A more detailed review of methods for analysing longitudinal data relevant to HTA, with particular emphasis on the implementation of methods is needed.

References

1. American Food and Drug Administration. *Guideline for the format and content of the clinical and statistical sections of new drug applications*, July 1988.
2. Committee on Proprietary Medicinal Products Working Party on Efficacy of Medicinal Products. Biostatistical methodology in clinical trials in applications for market for medicinal products. *Statist Med* 1995;**14**:1659–82.
3. Department of Health. *Briefing pack for research ethics committee members*, 1997. (Available from Department of Health, PO Box 410, LS23 7LL.)
4. International Conference on Harmonisation. *Structure and content of clinical study reports, November 1997*. (Note: Medicines Control Agency EuroDirect Publication No. 137/95.)
5. Joint Committee of MCA, ABPI, BMA, CSM and RCGP. *Guidelines for company-sponsored safety assessment of marketed medicines, November 1993*.
6. Statisticians in the Pharmaceutical Industry Professional Standards Working Party. *Guideline standard operating procedures for good statistical practice in clinical research, 1991, 1994*. (Note: Continually being reviewed and updated.)
7. Medical Research Council. *MRC ethics series, January 1995*. (Note: A series of six booklets.)

8. van Oortmarssen GJ, Boer R, Habbema JDF. Modelling issues in cancer screening. *Statist Methods Med Res* 1994;**3**:33–54.

9. Etzioni RD, Connor RJ, Prorok PC, Self SG. Design and analysis of cancer screening trials. *Statist Methods Med Res* 1994;**3**:3–17.

10. Enas G, Goldstein DJ. Defining, monitoring and combining safety information in clinical trials. *Statist Med* 1995;**14**:1099–111.

11. O'Neill RT. Statistical concepts in the planning and evaluation of drug safety from clinical trials in drug development: issues of international harmonization. *Statist Med* 1995;**14**:1117–27.

12. Zahl PH. A proportional regression model for 20 year survival of colon cancer in Norway. *Statist Med* 1995;**14**:1249–61.

13. Satten GA, Longini IM Jr. Markov chains with measurement error: estimating the "true" course of a marker of the progression of human immunodeficiency virus disease (with discussion). *Appl Statist* 1996;**45**:275–309.

14. Grubard BI, Korn EL. Regression analysis with clustered data. *Statist Med* 1994;**13**:509–22.

15. Raab GM, Gore SM, Goldberg DJ, Donnelly CA. Bayesian forecasting of the human immunodeficiency virus epidemic in Scotland. *Statist Society* 1994;**157**: 17–30.

16. Everitt BS. The analysis of repeated measures: a practical review with examples. *J Roy Statist Soc Series D* 1995;**44**:113–35.

14 An introduction to Bayesian methods in health services research

DAVID J SPIEGELHALTER,
JONATHAN P MYLES, DAVID R JONES
AND KEITH ABRAMS

Bayes theorem arose from a posthumous publication in 1763 by Thomas Bayes, a non-conformist minister from Tunbridge Wells. Although this publication described a simple and uncontroversial result in probability theory, specific uses of the theorem have been the subject of considerable controversy for over two centuries. In recent years a more balanced and pragmatic perspective has emerged, and in this chapter we review current thinking on the value of the Bayesian approach to health technology assessment (HTA).

A concise definition of Bayesian methods in HTA has not been established, but we suggest the following: *the explicit quantitative use of external evidence in the design, monitoring, analysis, interpretation and reporting in health technology assessment.*

A Bayesian perspective leads to an approach to clinical trials[1] that is claimed to be more flexible and ethical than traditional methods, and to elegant ways of handling multiple sub-studies, for example when simultaneously estimating the effects of a treatment on many subgroups.[2] Proponents have also argued that a Bayesian approach enables one to provide conclusions in a form that is most suitable for both patient-specific decisions and public policy.[3]

However, many questions remain, notably to what extent will the scientific community, or the regulatory authorities, allow the explicit consideration of evidence that is not totally derived from observed data? Here we outline the available literature, discuss the main techniques that are being suggested, and provide some recommendations for future work.

150

Nature of the evidence

A "Bayesian approach" can be applied to many scientific issues, and a search of the BIDS ISI database using this term yielded nearly 3500 papers over the period 1990–96. About 200 of these were relevant to HTA. Using these as a source for forward and backward searches, and searching other databases (Embase and MEDLINE) and sources, we identified about 300 papers, including around 50 reports of studies taking a fully Bayesian perspective. A considerable further number of studies have taken a so-called "empirical Bayes" approach, which uses elements of Bayesian modelling without giving a Bayesian interpretation to the conclusions; these are mentioned further below.

The published studies are dispersed throughout the literature, apart from one recent collection of papers.[4] The only textbook which might be considered to be on Bayesian methods in HTA focuses on the Confidence Profile Approach.[5] The studies are mainly demonstrations of the approach rather than complete assessments and, in spite of numerous articles advocating the use of Bayesian methods, practical take-up seems very low.

Findings

Philosophy of the Bayesian approach

Bayes' theorem is a formula which shows how existing beliefs, formally expressed as probability distributions, are modified by new information. The use of a diagnostic test is a familiar example of the type of situation to which it can be applied; a doctor's prior belief about whether a patient has a particular disease (based on knowledge of the prevalence of the disease in the community and the patient's symptoms) will be modified by the result of the test.[6]

Controversy arises when the unknown piece of information is a somewhat more intangible quantity than an individual's true diagnosis, such as the average effect of a drug on a particular group of patients. Such true underlying effects are not directly observable and are considered to be parameters: a Bayesian analyst is prepared to talk in terms of probabilities of parameter values and so say, for example, that "the chance is 15% that drug A improves survival over drug B". This type of statement is impossible to make within the traditional statistical framework, in which the interpretation of

Box 14.1 A Bayesian analysis of a hypothetical example

Suppose a randomised trial of the efficacy of a new cancer treatment has been carried out and a doctor has to decide whether to begin using the treatment routinely; the measure of efficacy to be used is the median increased months of survival of patients on the new treatment compared to the current treatment.

The most important difference between Bayesian and classical statistics is that the former allows an individual's opinion about the effectiveness of a treatment to be incorporated with the evidence from the study. The opinion is formally expressed as a "prior distribution" representing the strength of belief held by the individual for a range of plausible values of the quantity of interest. Suppose that, based on the doctor's knowledge of the disease and of the gains in efficacy of previous proposed new treatments, it is optimistically believed that the new treatment is most likely to increase median survival by about three months, but that there is a small probability that it either increases survival by more than 6 months or decreases it relative to the standard treatment (say 5% in either case). A possible prior distribution representing the doctor's beliefs is shown in Figure 14.1a, which shows that it is $0.22/0.12 = 1.8$ times more likely that the median increase in survival time is 3 months than 1 month. The shaded area shows the probability that is attached to the possibility that the new treatment reduces survival time, that is 5%.

The likelihood function expresses the plausibility of having observed the actual randomised trial data for different values of the "true" difference in median survival. For example, suppose the trial suggests a small improvement in survival of 1 month, but with considerable uncertainty; this is formally expressed by the likelihood function shown in Figure 14.1b, which shows that the trial data were $0.33/0.08 = 4.1$ times more likely to have arisen if the true increase in survival time were 1 month than 3 months.

Bayes' theorem generates a posterior distribution by multiplying the prior and the likelihood together for each value of the parameter of interest (and dividing the result by a constant to keep the area under the curve equal to 1). This represents the rational incorporation of the information from the randomised trial (the likelihood) with the doctor's prior belief (the prior distribution). The posterior distribution (Figure 14.1c) shows that the doctor (should) now believe that it is $0.33/0.15 = 2.2$ times more likely that the true median increase in survival time is 1 month than 3 months, and that the probability that the survival time is decreased by the new treatment is 5.5%. The doctor's belief about the relative probability of 1 month against 3 months' median improvement in survival has been strongly modified by the results of the trial, but the belief about the probability of a decrease in survival time has changed hardly at all.

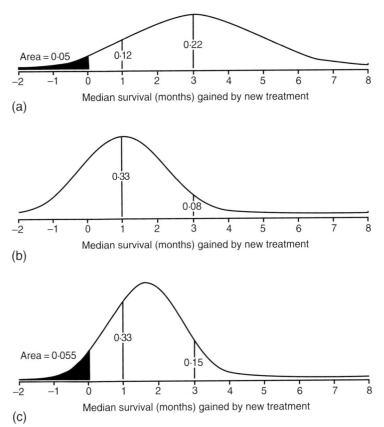

Figure 14.1. Prior (a), likelihood (b) and posterior (c) distributions arising from a hypothetical randomised trial. The relative prior, likelihood and posterior support for one and three months' survival are shown by the heights of the vertical lines, and the prior and posterior probabilities of a decrease in survival time are shown by the shaded areas.

P-values and confidence intervals depends on rather convoluted statements concerning the long-run properties of statistical procedures under null hypotheses. The use of Bayes' theorem in a simple hypothetical example is illustrated in Box 14.1, in which a doctor's "prior" distribution concerning the efficacy of a treatment is modified to a "posterior" distribution after observing some randomised trial data.

Table 14.1 briefly summarises some major distinctions between the Bayesian and the traditional approach. The latter is sometimes

Table 14.1   A brief comparison of Bayesian and frequentist methods in
randomised trials

Issue	Frequentist	Bayesian
Information other than that in the study being analysed	Informally used in design	Used formally by specifying a prior probability distribution
Interpretation of the parameter of interest	A fixed state of nature	An unknown quantity which can have a probability distribution
Basic question	"How likely is the data given a particular value of the parameter?"	"How likely is a particular value of the parameter given the data?"
Presentation of results	Likelihood functions, P-values, confidence intervals	Plots of posterior distributions of the parameter, calculation of specific posterior probabilities of interest, and use of the posterior distribution in formal decision analysis
Interim analyses	P-values and estimates adjusted for the number of analyses	Inference not affected by the number or timing of interim analyses
Interim predictions	Conditional power analyses	Predictive probability of getting a firm conclusion
Dealing with subsets in trials	Adjusted P-values (e.g. Bonferroni)	Subset effects shrunk towards zero by a "sceptical" prior

termed "frequentist" as it is based on the long-run frequency
properties of statistical procedures. There are many papers
summarising the Bayesian philosophy and its application to
randomised trials. Cornfield is a notable early example,[7] and others
have argued for the flexibility, coherence and intuitiveness of the
approach.[1-3,8] A number of authors have highlighted how the
Bayesian approach leads naturally into a formal decision theoretic
approach to randomised trials.[9]

Quantifying prior beliefs

The Bayesian approach is most controversial when there is no hard
evidence for the prior distribution, and we have to rely on subjective
judgement. This considerably broadens the area of potential
application, although the reasonableness of the judgements will
need to be justified. The traditional terms "prior" and "posterior"

may also be misleading, giving the impression that the prior has to be fixed before the evidence is examined. It is more helpful to think of the prior as summarising all external evidence about the quantity of interest, for example other published studies, which might arise during or after the study being considered.

One source of a prior distribution is the pooled subjective opinion of informed experts, which can be elicited interactively using computer programs[10] or using questionnaire methods.[11] Another source is meta-analyses of previous similar studies. One important use of a prior distribution is in planning the sample size of a randomised trial. Instead of the use of a single (possibly optimistic) alternative hypothesis as the basis for the power calculation, the prior distribution can be used to produce an "expected power", with reasonable uncertainty about the true treatment effect taken into account.[11]

There has been an increasing move towards "off-the-shelf" priors, specifically those of a sceptic and an enthusiast,[12] to represent extreme opinions in sensitivity analyses; they can also be used in sequential monitoring of trials (see below). One published example concerns the use of sceptical priors in determining whether there is sufficient evidence for a treatment to be generally recommended (Box 14.2).

Applications in monitoring randomised trials

Using the traditional frequentist approach, randomised trials are designed to have a fixed chance (usually 5%) of incorrectly rejecting the null hypothesis, and a variety of techniques have been developed for adjusting the apparent significance level of a result to allow for the fact that the data have been analysed more than once. The Bayesian approach sees no need for this, and instead monitors the trial on the basis of the current posterior distribution, providing an updated summary of the evidence about the treatment effect at the time of any analysis. Several monitoring schemes have been suggested, some of which are based on decision theory.[9] However, the most frequently illustrated is simply based on the "tail" areas of the posterior distribution: for example, stop the trial if the chance that the treatment is more effective than control is greater than 99%.[14] If desired, the probability of the treatment effect being greater than some clinically important difference may be used, or,

Box 14.2 Bayes' theorem in a randomised trial

Parmar et al.[13] illustrate the use of a sceptical prior distribution in deciding whether or not to perform a confirmatory randomised trial. They discuss a Cancer and Leukaemia Group B (CALGB) trial of radiotherapy and chemotherapy versus standard radiotherapy in patients with locally advanced stage III non-small cell lung cancer. This trial showed an adjusted median improvement in survival of 6·3 months (95% confidence interval 1·4 to 13·3 months) in favour of the new treatment, which has a two-sided P-value of 0·008. They suggest two arguments why this might not lead to an immediate recommendation for radiotherapy and chemotherapy as standard treatment. First, the toxicity of chemotherapy might mean a minimum worthwhile improvement is demanded, and they suggest a figure of around four months. Second, a natural scepticism exists about new cancer therapies, derived from long experience of failed innovations.

These two aspects can be formalised within the Bayesian framework. First, one can report the probability that the new treatment not only provides a positive improvement, but that this exceeds a minimum clinically worthwhile improvement. Second, scepticism is expressed by a prior distribution centred on zero improvement, and which shows a 5% chance that the true improvement is greater than the alternative hypothesis in this study, namely that the true improvement is five months.

Figure 14.2 shows this sceptical prior distribution, which provides equivalent evidence to an "imaginary" trial in which 33 patients died on each treatment. The dashed vertical lines display the null hypothesis of no improvement and the minimum clinically worthwhile improvement of 4 months. Between these lie what can be termed the "range of equivalence", and the figure shows that the sceptical prior expresses a probability of 41% that the true benefit lies in the range of equivalence, and only 9% that the new treatment is clinically superior.

The likelihood function shows the inferences to be made from the data alone, assuming a "uniform" prior on the range of possible improvements; Parmar et al. call this an "enthusiastic" prior. The probability that the new treatment is actually inferior is 0·4% (equivalent to the one-sided P-value of 0·008/2). The probability of clinical superiority is 80%, which might be considered sufficient to change treatment policy.

The posterior distribution shows the impact of the sceptical prior, in that the chance of clinical superiority is reduced to 44%, hardly sufficient to change practice. In fact, Parmar et al. report that the NCI Intergroup Trial investigators were unconvinced by the CALGB trial because of their previous negative experience, and so carried out a further study. They found a significant median improvement but of only 2·4 months, suggesting the sceptical approach might have given a more reasonable estimate.

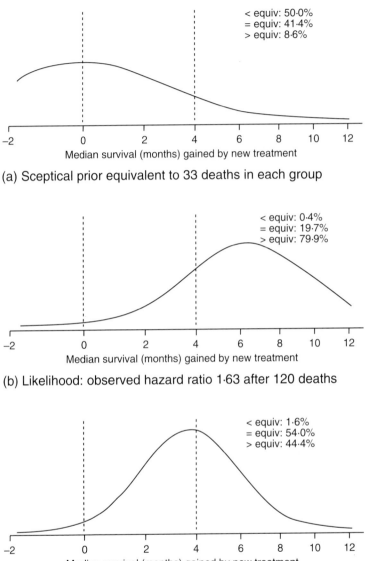

< equiv: 50·0%
= equiv: 41·4%
> equiv: 8·6%

(a) Sceptical prior equivalent to 33 deaths in each group

< equiv: 0·4%
= equiv: 19·7%
> equiv: 79·9%

(b) Likelihood: observed hazard ratio 1·63 after 120 deaths

< equiv: 1·6%
= equiv: 54·0%
> equiv: 44·4%

(c) Posterior distribution

Figure 14.2. Prior, likelihood and posterior distributions arising from CALGB trial of standard radiotherapy versus additional chemotherapy in advanced lung cancer.[13] The dashed lines give the boundaries of the range of clinical equivalence, taken to be 0 to 4 months median improvement in survival. Numbers by each graph show the probabilities of lying below, within and above the range of equivalence.

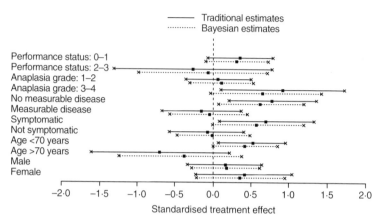

Figure 14.3. Traditional and Bayesian estimates of standardised treatment effects in a cancer randomised trial. The Bayesian estimates are pulled towards the overall treatment effect by a degree determined by the empirical heterogeneity of the subset results.

in the case of equivalence studies, that the treatment difference is less than, say, 10%.

If a sceptical prior is used, the trial data must overcome a handicap. Hence the approach shows conservatism in the light of early positive results, which can be remarkably similar to that of frequentist stopping rules.[15] The use of sceptical priors has been described in a tutorial[16] and in meta-analyses.[17] A senior statistician with the US Food and Drug Administration has said that he "would like to see [sceptical priors] applied in more routine fashion to provide insight into our decision making."[18]

Table 14.1 also considers predictions made at an interim stage in a randomised trial. Whereas the frequentist conditional power calculations are based on a hypothesised value of the true treatment effect, a Bayesian approach can answer the crucial question: if we continue the study, what is the chance we will get a significant result?

Multiplicity – estimating the prior

We often wish simultaneously to carry out a set of related analyses, for example meta-analysis of individual trial results, allowing for between-centre variability in the analysis of a multicentre trial, or analysing subsets of cases in a single trial. We call these "sub-studies". The traditional frequentist approach tries to maintain a constant probability of wrongly rejecting the null hypothesis (Type I error) by some adjustment, for example a Bonferroni method for multiple comparisons.

The Bayesian approach integrates subanalyses by assuming that the unknown quantities (for example, the subset-specific treatment effects) have a common prior distribution, with the important difference that this prior distribution has unknown parameters that need to be estimated. Such models are known as hierarchical and can, in theory, have any number of levels, although three is generally enough. Non-Bayesian versions exist, known as multilevel, random effects and random coefficient models, which use either likelihood or "empirical Bayes" approaches to estimate the model parameters.

In general, the priors have a "sceptical" form, postulating that differences between subanalyses are limited. The degree of homogeneity observed between the sub-studies is used to estimate their prior similarity, for example the between-trial variability in a meta-analysis. Both full Bayesian and empirical Bayes approaches can lead to similar conservatism.[19] An example is shown in Box 14.3.

Non-randomised studies and evidence synthesis

Most authors have concentrated on the application of Bayesian methods when designing randomised trials or pooling results from published trials, but a small number of papers have considered their application to data collected from non-randomised studies. For example, in a paper analysing data from two case-control studies (one being very small) and a cohort study,[21] the authors show the results of using different sources of information for the prior and likelihood. Other authors have discussed the integration of evidence from a number of different types of non-randomised studies,[22] and the integration of findings from both randomised and non-randomised studies within a Bayesian framework.[23,24]

Decision-making

Another important feature of a Bayesian approach is the way in which the resulting posterior probability distribution can be combined with quantitative measures of utility as part of a formal decision analysis.[25] As with the elicitation of beliefs regarding probabilities, the elicitation and quantification of utilities is challenging, and is one of the least developed areas of Bayesian

---

Box 14.3 Bayes' theorem for subset analysis

Dixon and Simon[20] describe a Bayesian approach to dealing with subset analysis in a randomised trial in advanced colorectal cancer. The solid horizontal lines in Figure 14.3 show the standardised treatment effects within a range of subgroups, using traditional methods for estimating treatment by subgroup interactions. Four of the 12 intervals exclude zero, although due to the multiple hypotheses being tested an adjustment technique such as Bonferroni might be used to decrease the apparent statistical significance of these findings.

The Bayesian approach is to assume subgroup-specific deviations from the overall treatment effect have a prior distribution centred at zero but with an unknown variability; this variability is then given its own prior distribution. Since the degree of scepticism is governed by the variance of the prior distribution, the observed heterogeneity of treatment effects between subgroups will influence the degree of scepticism being imposed.

The resulting Bayesian estimates are shown as dashed lines in Figure 14.3. They tend to be pulled towards each other, because of the prior scepticism about substantial subgroup-by-treatment interaction effects. Only one 95% confidence interval now excludes zero, the subgroup with no measurable metastatic disease. Dixon and Simon mention that this was the conclusion of the original trial, but that the Bayesian analysis has the advantage of not relying on somewhat arbitrary adjustment techniques, being generalisable to any number of subsets, and provides a unified means of both providing estimates and tests of hypotheses.

---

analysis. Decision theoretic methods have been applied in HTA in a variety of settings, including the development of clinical recommendations for prevention of stroke,[26] monitoring and analysis in randomised trials,[9] and assessment of environmental contamination on public health.[27]

Recommendations

Bayesian analysis is widely used in a variety of non-medical fields, including engineering, image-processing, expert systems, decision analysis, gene finding, financial predictions, and neural networks. There is also increasing use of Bayesian methods in complex epidemiological models. HTA has been slow to adopt Bayesian methods, which could be due to a reluctance to use prior opinions, unfamiliarity, mathematical complexity, lack of software, or conservatism of the health care establishment and, in particular, the regulatory authorities.

There are strong philosophical reasons for using a Bayesian approach, but the current literature emphasises the practical advantages in handling complex interrelated problems, and in making explicit and accountable what is usually implicit and hidden, thereby clarifying discussions and disagreements. The most persuasive reason is that the analysis tells us what we want to know: how should this piece of evidence change what we currently believe?

There are a number of perceived problems with the Bayesian approach, largely concerning the source of the prior and the interpretations of the conclusions. There are also practical difficulties in implementation and software. Although the current European guidelines for statistical submissions for drug regulatory authorities state that "the use of Bayesian or other well-argued approaches is quite acceptable",[28] it seems sensible that experience be gained in the use of Bayesian approaches in HTA in parallel with traditional approaches, and in such a way as to facilitate examination of the sensitivity of results to prior distributions.

Our recommendations for future practical methodological developments are:

1. An extended set of case studies showing practical aspects of the Bayesian approach, in particular for prediction and handling multiple sub-studies, in which mathematical details are minimised.
2. The development of standards for the performance and reporting of Bayesian analyses.[29]
3. The development and dissemination of software for Bayesian analysis, preferably as part of existing packages.

References

1. Kadane JB. Prime time for Bayes. *Controlled Clin Trials* 1995;**16**:313–18.
2. Breslow N. Biostatistics and Bayes. *Statist Sci* 1990;**5**:269–84.
3. Lilford RJ, Braunholtz D. For debate – the statistical basis of public-policy – a paradigm shift is overdue. *Br Med J* 1996;**313**:603–7.
4. Berry DA, Stangl DK. *Bayesian biostatistics*. New York: Marcel Dekker, 1996.
5. Eddy DM, Hasselblad V, Shachter R. *Meta-analysis by the confidence profile method: the statistical synthesis of evidence*. San Diego, CA: Academic Press, 1992.
6. Sackett DL, Haynes RB, Guyatt GH, Tugwell P. *Clinical epidemiology: a basic science for clinical medicine* Boston, MA: Little Brown, 2nd edn, 1991.

7. Cornfield J. Recent methodological contributions to clinical trials. *Am J Epidemiol* 1976;**104**:408–21.
8. Lewis RJ, Wears RL. An introduction to the Bayesian analysis of clinical trials. *Ann Emergency Med* 1993;**22**:1328–36.
9. Berry DA, Wolff MC, Sack D. Decision-making during a Phase-III randomized controlled trial. *Controlled Clin Trials* 1994;**15**:360–78.
10. Chaloner K, Church T, Louis TA, Matts JP. Graphical elicitation of a prior distribution for a clinical-trial. *Statistician* 1993;**42**:341–53.
11. Parmar MKB, Spiegelhalter DJ, Freedman LS *et al*. The Chart trials: Bayesian design and monitoring in practice. *Statist Med* 1994;**13**:1297–312.
12. Spiegelhalter DJ, Freedman LS, Parmar MKB. Bayesian approaches to randomized trials. *J Roy Statist Soc Series A* 1994;**157**:357–87.
13. Parmar MKB, Ungerleider RS, Simon R. Assessing whether to perform a confirmatory randomized clinical-trial. *J Nat Cancer Inst* 1996;**88**:1645–51.
14. Freedman LS, Spiegelhalter DJ, Parmar MKB. The what, why and how of Bayesian clinical-trials monitoring. *Statist Med* 1994;**13**:1371–83.
15. Grossman J, Parmar MKB, Spiegelhalter DJ, Freedman LS. A unified method for monitoring and analysing controlled trials. *Statist Med* 1994;**13**:1815–26.
16. Fayers PM, Ashby D, Parmar MKB. Bayesian data monitoring in clinical trials. *Statist Med* 1997;**16**:1413–30.
17. Dersimonian R. Metaanalysis in the design and monitoring of clinical-trials. Statist Med 1996;**15**:1237–48.
18. O'Neill R. Early stopping rules workshop: conclusions. *Statist Med* 1994;**13**: 1493–9.
19. Louis TA. Using empirical Bayes methods in biopharmaceutical research. *Statist Med* 1991;**10**:811–29.
20. Dixon DO, Simon R. Bayesian subset analysis in a colorectal cancer clinical trial. *Statist Med* 1992;**11**:13–22.
21. Ashby D, Hutton J, McGee M. Simple Bayesian analyses for case-control studies in cancer epidemiology. *Statistician* 1993;**42**:385–97.
22. Eddy DM, Hasselblad V, Shachter R. An introduction to a Bayesian method for meta-analysis – the confidence profile method. *Med Decision Making* 1990; **10**:15–23.
23. Abrams KR, Jones DR. Meta-analysis and the synthesis of evidence. *IMA J Math Med Biol* 1995;**12**:297–313.
24. Smith TC, Abrams KR, Jones DR. Hierarchical models in generalised synthesis of evidence: an example based on studies of breast cancer screening. *Tech Rep 95-02*, 1995. Department of Epidemiology and Public Health, University of Leicester.
25. Smith JQ. *Decision analysis – a Bayesian approach*. London; Chapman and Hall, 1988.
26. Parmigiani G, Ancukiewicz M, Matchar D. Decision models in clinical recommendations development: the stroke prevention policy model. In: Berry A, Stangl DK (eds), *Bayesian biostatistics*. New York: Marcel Dekker, 1996.
27. Wolfson LJ, Kadane JD, Small MJ. Expected utility as a policy-making tool: an environmental health example. In: Berry A, Stangl DK (eds), *Bayesian biostatistics*. New York: Marcel Dekker, 1996.
28. Lewis JA, Jones DR, Roehmel J. Biostatistical methodology in clinical trials – a European guideline. *Statist Med* 1995;**14**:1655–8.
29. Spiegelhalter DJ, Myles J, Jones DR, Abrams KR. Bayesian methods in health technology assessment. *Health Technol Assess* (in press).

15 Quality of life assessment and survival data

LUCINDA J BILLINGHAM, KEITH ABRAMS
AND DAVID R JONES

Quality of life has become an important issue in health care, especially in studies of interventions for chronic diseases where halting or slowing progression, rather than cure, is the aim. Substantial amounts of quality of life data are now being gathered in clinical studies using specially developed instruments.[1] In studies which assess both quality of life and survival, patients are generally severely ill and it is a common occurrence for participants to drop out of the quality of life study due to illness or death. In these situations, the dropout process may depend on the quality of life being experienced, rather than being random. The incomplete follow-up of patients is called *informative dropout*. The relationship between dropout and quality of life needs to be accounted for appropriately in any analysis of the data otherwise it could introduce bias.

This chapter describes methods that have been proposed for the assessment of health technologies with respect to their effect on both quality and length of life, particularly those that simultaneously assess these two endpoints. The aim was to identify methods that require wider dissemination and areas that require further research.

Nature of the evidence

Scientific and medical literature were searched for relevant methodological articles. Electronic searches using BIDS (Bath Information and Data Service) databases were supplemented by exploded references, personal collections, and a hand search of the journal *Quality of Life Research*.

Methods for analysing quality of life and survival data were found to fall into three broad categories according to the research question underlying the study.

- Methods for studies where the primary aim is to compare treatments in terms of their effect on quality of life whilst accounting for informative dropout.
- Methods for studies that primarily aim to compare the length of survival conferred by different treatments whilst adjusting for the effects of quality of life.
- Methods for studies where quality of life and survival are both important endpoints for assessing treatments, and the two endpoints are analysed simultaneously.

This last category forms the main body of literature from the review and the chapter focuses on this area.

Findings

Quality of life assessment in the presence of informative dropout

The analysis of longitudinal quality of life data should begin descriptively, with the use of plots of individual patient profiles and group profiles, to give insight into the data before any formal testing or modelling is carried out.[2,3] An initial approach to the analysis is to use summary measures,[4] where treatment comparison is based on a single value summarising the quality of life data over time. However, not only will informative dropout probably still cause a problem (depending on the summary measure that is chosen), but also the method does not capture the dynamic nature of quality of life data.

Longitudinal quality of life data can be modelled using methods such as repeated measures analysis of variance, or more complex techniques such as random coefficient models and marginal models.[5] The application of these methods to quality of life data with missing measurements has been discussed.[3,6–8] Although these techniques model change over time, they assume missing data are missing at random and may therefore give biased results when informative dropout is present. Modelling techniques that deal with informative dropout have been developed[9,10] but examples of their application to quality of life data are limited.

Assessment of survival data adjusting for quality of life

When the length of survival for different treatments is being compared, it is often necessary to adjust for other patient-related factors, known as covariates, that could potentially affect the survival time of a patient.[11,12] In some situations the survival analysis may need to adjust for baseline measures of quality of life (fixed covariates), whilst in others adjustments for changes in quality of life over time may be required (time-dependent covariates). If assessments of quality of life are infrequent or data are missing for reasons other than death, then it may be difficult to adjust for changing quality of life with any degree of accuracy.

Simultaneous assessment of quality of life and survival

In studies where quality of life and survival are both important endpoints, it may be advantageous to assess health technologies in terms of these endpoints simultaneously. Three different approaches can be used to achieve this.

- Quality-adjusted survival analysis compares treatments in terms of a composite measure of quality and quantity of life, created by weighting periods of survival time according to the quality of life experienced.
- Multistate survival analysis describes the movement of patients through various health states defined by levels of quality of life and death, and explores how treatments differ in terms of these movements.
- Simultaneous modelling is a complex statistical approach that considers quality of life and survival as two simultaneous processes and describes the data in terms of two interlinked models.

There is some controversy regarding the simultaneous analysis of quality of life and survival data. One view is that the time-dependent structure of the individual quality of life process can best be accounted for when quality and quantity of survival are analysed simultaneously,[13] whilst another is that methods which

165

attempt to combine quality of life and survival into a single measure are generally inappropriate.[14,15] It may be preferable in certain situations to analyse and report quality of life and survival outcomes separately, so that any conflict between the two with respect to the treatment comparison is apparent.[16]

Quality-adjusted survival analysis

Quality and quantity of life can be combined into a single endpoint by weighting periods of survival time according to the quality of life experienced during these periods. The weights typically have the properties of utilities[17] and range from 0 to 1, where 0 represents quality of life equivalent to death and 1 represents perfect health; negative weights can be used to represent a quality of life worse than death. The resulting outcome is generally measured in Quality-Adjusted Life Years (QALYs).[18]

Special forms of QALYs are TWiST (Time Without Symptoms or Toxicity)[19,20] and Q-TWiST (Quality-adjusted TWiST).[21,22] For TWiST, all periods of survival time with symptoms of disease or toxicity resulting from treatment are given a weight of 0 whilst all other time periods are given a weight of 1 so that, as its name suggests, TWiST only counts time without symptoms or toxicity. The Q-TWiST endpoint is a more general form of TWiST where periods of survival time spent with symptoms of disease and toxicity resulting from treatment are each given a weight between 0 and 1, rather than being ignored as they are in TWiST (Box 15.1).

If survival times are known for all patients in a study (that is, none are censored) and quality of life for the full duration of survival is known, QALYs can be calculated for all subjects and treatment comparison is straightforward. It is more usual, however, for some survival times to be censored. Again, QALYs can be calculated for each subject and standard survival analysis techniques may seem appropriate. There is, however, informative censoring because subjects with worse quality of life will be censored earlier than those with good quality of life, and this will bias the results.[18]

One attempt to solve the problem is to restrict the analysis to a time period, chosen to reduce (or ideally eliminate) censored data. This may be impractical if some survival times are censored early. The most widely used method is partitioned survival analysis[18,23] where overall survival time is partitioned into time spent in a series of progressive health states (Box 15.2 and Figure 15.1). The main limitation of partitioned survival analysis is the need to use

---

Box 15.1 Example of Q-TWiST in breast cancer

Goldhirsch et al.[21] considered evaluating the use of adjuvant therapy for post-menopausal node-positive breast cancer patients in terms of a Q-TWiST endpoint. The overall survival time for each patient was divided into three possible periods on the basis of whether or not either treatment-related toxicity or symptoms of disease progression were experienced. In addition to adjuvant therapy resulting in improved overall survival, it was also shown to be superior in terms of Q-TWiST assuming weights of 0.5 for periods of toxicity and periods of disease progression, relative to a weight of 1.0 for TWiST. A sensitivity analysis revealed that provided the weight assigned to periods with toxicity was greater than that assigned to periods of disease progression, then adjuvant therapy was to be preferred.

Box 15.2 Example of partitioned survival analysis in lung cancer

Billingham et al.[30] consider the use of partitioned survival analysis to evaluate the use of chemotherapy, compared to palliation, in patients with advanced non-small cell lung cancer over an 18-week treatment period. Overall survival during this time was partitioned into four progressive health states depending on whether, and when, "poor" quality of life, as defined by responses to a quality of life instrument, was experienced. Figure 15.1 displays graphically the time spent in each of the four health states for patients on the chemotherapy arm of the trial. A sensitivity analysis revealed that regardless of the choice of weights for the two "poor" health states, compared to a weight of 1.0 for the "good" health states, chemotherapy appeared to be beneficial.

---

progressive health states, which may not always be easy to define or clinically relevant. A parametric approach to quality-adjusted survival analysis may overcome some of the limitations of the method.[24]

Often quality of life is recorded only for a limited amount of survival time, for example one year from study entry, and the comparison of treatments in terms of quality-adjusted survival is then restricted to that time period. There is no unique way to divide the survival time of patients into periods of differing quality

167

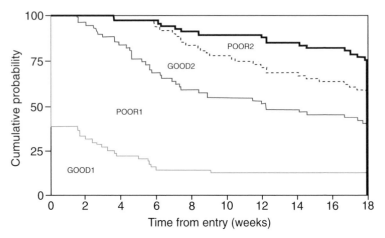

Figure 15.1   Example of partitioned survival analysis (see Box 15.2).

of life, and the accuracy depends on the frequency of quality of life assessments. Different divisions need to be considered as part of a sensitivity analysis. Missing quality of life data will also cause difficulties since, although quality-adjusted survival analysis deals with informative dropout from death, it does not deal with other reasons for dropout. It may be possible to impute values for missing data; otherwise a method that explicitly models the dropout process should be considered.

Multistate survival analysis
An alternative approach to quality-adjusted survival analysis is multistate survival analysis. Although multistate models have been advocated and discussed as a possible means of analysing quality of life and survival data simultaneously,[13,14] there is little evidence of their application in this field.

Multistate survival analysis starts by categorising the follow-up time of patients in a trial into a number of different health states, including death. Definitions of these health states in terms of quality of life data, and the possible transitions between them constitute the multistate model. The simplest version is a three-state illness-death model where there are two transient "alive" states: "alive without illness" and "alive with illness", and one absorbing "death" state (Figure 15.2).

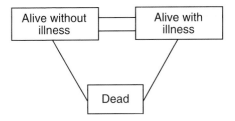

Figure 15.2   A three-state illness/death model.

The movement between health states is described by transition rates which are modelled using the transition times for patients. If the exact transition times are known, standard semi- and fully-parametric models can be used.[25] Alternatively, if all that is known for a patient is the health state occupied at each follow-up time, the transition rates can be modelled using a general continuous-time Markov chain.[26]

As with quality-adjusted survival analysis, different definitions of health states need to be considered as part of a sensitivity analysis, and the accuracy of the transition times depends on the frequency of quality of life assessments. The inclusion of death as a health state in the model enables the analysis to deal with informative dropout from death. Informative dropout for other reasons can be dealt with either by imputing values for the missing data or by including a "dropout" health state in the model.

Quality of life and survival as two simultaneous processes
Longitudinal quality of life data can be modelled simultaneously with the dropout process, which includes dropout from death.[27] The simultaneous modelling of repeatedly measured covariates and survival data has been described,[28,29] but has not been applied to quality of life data. Such an approach has the advantage of allowing quality of life data to be assessed longitudinally whilst adjusting for informative dropout. In addition the interrelationship between the two can be explored.

Recommendations

A critical review of the methods proposed for the analysis of quality of life and survival data together with their application to data from a previously conducted study[30] has given rise to the following recommendations for practitioners and researchers.

1. The method of analysis needs to be considered at the design stage of a study so that appropriate quality of life data can be collected. Issues to be considered are:

   - the quality of life instrument to be used;
   - the frequency and timing of quality of life assessments;
   - the need to minimise non-compliance;
   - the collection of additional information such as reasons for dropout; and
   - the sample size required.

2. The choice of method should be based on the research question that the study aims to answer. The advantages and disadvantages of each method should be considered together with the relevance and interpretability of the results to clinicians and patients.

3. Methods used to analyse longitudinal quality of life data must allow for informative dropout.

4. Methods used should be reported clearly, with details of definitions and assumptions used in the analysis.

5. Sensitivity analysis should be carried out to assess the robustness of conclusions to any critical assumptions made in the analysis.

6. Further experience in the application of quality-adjusted survival analysis techniques to quality of life data is needed to enable a proper evaluation of such methods.

7. Further research is needed to develop hierarchical models, multistate models, and simultaneous modelling methods in their practical application to quality of life and survival data with the use of both classical and Bayesian approaches. Consideration should be given as to how methods could deal with the multivariate nature of the quality of life endpoint.

8. A full review of available software for methods that simultaneously assess quality of life and survival data is needed to highlight areas requiring further development.

References

1. Bowling A. *Measuring health: a review of quality of life measurement scales.* Buckingham: Open University Press, 1991.

2. Fayers PM, Jones DR. Measuring and analysing quality of life in cancer clinical trials: a review. *Statist Med* 1983;2:429–46.
3. Beacon HJ. *The statistical analysis of self-assessed quality of life data in cancer clinical trials.* Thesis, University of London, 1996.
4. Matthews JNS, Altman DG, Campbell MJ, Royston P. Analysis of serial measurements in medical research. *Br Med J* 1990;300:230–5.
5. Diggle PJ, Liang K, Zeger SL. *Analysis of longitudinal data.* Oxford: Clarendon Press, 1994.
6. Zwinderman AH. Statistical analysis of longitudinal quality of life data with missing measurements. *Qual Life Res* 1992;1:219–24.
7. Zwinderman AH. The measurement of change of quality of life in clinical trials. *Statist Med* 1990;9:931–42.
8. Beacon HJ, Thompson S. Multi-level models for repeated measurement data: application to quality of life data in clinical trials. *Statist Med* 1996;15:2717–32.
9. De Stavola BL, Christensen E. Multilevel models for longitudinal variables prognostic for survival. *Lifetime Data Anal* 1996;2:329–47.
10. Little RJA. Modelling the drop-out mechanism in repeated measures studies. *J Am Statist Assoc* 1995;90:1112–21.
11. Collett D. *Modelling survival data in medical research.* London: Chapman and Hall, 1994.
12. Cox DR. Regression models and life tables. *J Roy Statist Soc B* 1972;34: 187–220.
13. Olschewski M, Schumacher M. Statistical analysis of quality of life data in cancer clinical trials. *Statist Med* 1990;9:749–63.
14. Cox DR, Fitzpatrick R, Fletcher AE, Gore SM, Spiegelhalter DJ, Jones DR. Quality-of-life assessment: can we keep it simple. *J Roy Statist Soc A:* 1992; 155:353–93.
15. Hopwood P, Stephens RJ, Machin D. Approaches to the analysis of quality of life data: experiences gained from a Medical Research Council Lung Cancer Working Party palliative chemotherapy trial. *Qual Life Res* 1994;3:339–52.
16. Fletcher A, Gore SM, Jones DR, Fitzpatrick R, Spiegelhalter DJ, Cox DR. Quality of life measures in health care. II: Design, analysis and interpretation. *Br Med J* 1992;305:1145–8.
17. Torrance GW. Utility approach to measuring health-related quality of life. *J Chronic Dis* 1987;40:593–600.
18. Glasziou PP, Simes RJ, Gelber RD. Quality adjusted survival analysis. *Statist Med* 1990;9:1259–76.
19. Gelber RD, Goldhirsch A. A new endpoint for the assessment of adjuvant therapy in postmenopausal women with operable breast cancer. *J Clin Oncol* 1986;4:1772–9.
20. Gelber RD, Gelman RS, Goldhirsch A. A quality-of-life-oriented endpoint for comparing therapies. *Biometrics* 1989; 45:781–95.
21. Goldhirsch A, Gelber RD, Simes RJ, Glasziou P, Coates AS. Costs and benefits of adjuvant therapy in breast-cancer: a quality-adjusted survival analysis. *J Clin Oncol* 1989;7:36–44.
22. Gelber RD, Cole BF, Gelber S, Goldhirsch A. Comparing treatments using quality-adjusted survival: the Q-TWiST method. *Am Statist* 1995;49:161–9.
23. Cole BF, Gelber RD, Goldhirsch A. Cox regression-models for quality-adjusted survival analysis. *Statist Med* 1993;12:975–87.
24. Cole BF, Gelber RD, Anderson KM. Parametric approaches to quality-adjusted survival analysis. *Biometrics* 1994;50:621–31.
25. Kay R. The analysis of transition times in multistate stochastic processes using proportional hazard regression models. *Commun Statist – Theory Methodol* 1982; 11:1743–56.

26. Kay R. A Markov model for analysing cancer markers and disease states in survival studies. *Biometrics* 1986;**42**:855–65.
27. Lindsey JK. *Modelling longitudinal measurement dropouts as a survival process with time-varying covariates*. Technical Report, Belgium: Limburgs Universitair Centrum, 1997.
28. Faucett CL, Thomas DC. Simultaneously modelling censored survival data and repeatedly measured covariates: a Gibbs sampling approach. *Statist Med* 1996;**15**:1663–85.
29. Berzuini C. Medical monitoring. In: Gilks WR, Richardson S, Spiegelhalter DJ (eds), *Markov chain Monte Carlo in practice*. London: Chapman and Hall, 1995.
30. Billingham LJ, Abrams KR, Jones DR. Quality of life assessment and survival data. *Health Technol Assess* 1998 (in press).

Part Four
Presenting, interpreting, and synthesising evidence

16 Systematic reviews of randomised trials

ALEXANDER J SUTTON, DAVID R JONES,
KEITH ABRAMS, TREVOR A SHELDON
AND FUJIAN SONG

Systematic reviews and meta-analytical methods are now commonly used approaches to the assessment of health care interventions and the increasing adoption of such techniques is likely, partly in response to the emphasis on "evidence-based" approaches to health care and also the explosion of publications beyond the capacity of all, except specialist, researchers. If a set of studies investigating a common intervention is such that it is appropriate to combine them, synthesis of their results may yield a more precise estimate of the treatment/policy benefit, and perhaps also reduce the bias associated with specific individual studies. Additionally, combining several sources of evidence may increase the generalisability of the results and allow a full exploration of the effects in subgroups. More importantly, adopting the rigorous methods required to carry out a systematic review can highlight deficiencies in the existing literature, or methodological differences between studies, and inform future research priorities.

Meta-analysis has come a long way since its inception and has matured to the extent that several sets of guidelines concerning at least the basics of the review process have been published.[1-4] However, several contentious issues remain unresolved, and methods are currently inadequate in certain instances. This chapter has three aims:

- to summarise the methods for systematic reviews and meta-analyses in health technology assessment;
- to promote the appropriate use of such approaches; and

- to highlight areas where further methodological development is required.

Nature of the evidence

The relevant methodological literature is already substantial. We identified approximately 1000 potentially relevant references, including some from educational research, psychology, and sociology.[5] Methods for systematic reviews encompass many topics from prereview issues, such as methods of literature searching, through mainstream methods of description and synthesis, to the dissemination of the review's findings. The literature reflects this diversity. A considerable body of work exists on the statistical aspects of combining, or meta-analysing, study results, with increasingly sophisticated methods being developed over time. A brief resumé of the general statistical methods available for formally combining several study estimates is given below. The reader should be aware that other methods specific to various outcome measures and data types, not discussed here, also exist.[5]

Findings

Procedures

The procedures necessary for carrying out all stages of a systematic review have been clearly defined in two sets of guidelines.[1,2] Our recommendations for systematic review practice at the end of this chapter build on these. From investigations into the effectiveness of different search methods,[6] it would appear that researchers should use several approaches, such as database searching complemented by hand searching of key journals. All searches carried out must be documented sufficiently in order to allow others to replicate them.

Quality of primary research studies

It is common to assess the quality of the primary studies eligible for inclusion in the review. Exclusion of poor quality studies, or at least a downweighting of them in a formal pooled analysis, may appear sensible, but no consensus has been reached as to the best way to proceed. The problem stems largely from the fact that although many scales for scoring the quality of randomised trials[7] and other studies exist,[8] there is little evidence regarding the validity of these instruments. Indeed, it is difficult to justify any cut-off value for the exclusion of studies, or weighting of studies by the quality scores, because they are often constructed in an arbitrary way. An alternative procedure is to consider a reduced set of components associated with study quality, and explore the effect of each one separately. Whichever approach is adopted, a sensitivity analysis of the impact on the subsequent decisions made is essential.

Heterogeneity

Heterogeneity refers to the variation that may be found between studies in the estimates of the effectiveness of an intervention, above that expected by sampling error alone. Heterogeneity has both advantages and disadvantages; exploring reasons for its presence can lead to useful clinical insights, while accounting for it can make modelling problematic. If heterogeneity is extremely large, combining study estimates may be rejected on the grounds that any overall estimate makes little sense. Pooling study estimates when there is a strong possibility of heterogeneity requires an appropriate analysis which explains, or accounts for it. Models for doing this are discussed below. Generally, no consensus has been reached concerning the best strategy for dealing with heterogeneity.

Combining treatment estimates

A series of different methods of increasing sophistication has been developed for the pooling of estimates from primary studies. The simplest include vote counting, where the number of studies showing beneficial and harmful effects are tallied. Alternatively the combination of P-values of the treatment effect for each study has also been advocated. Neither method yields a pooled estimate of effect size and both can only be recommended as a last resort when, owing to limitations in information available from study reports, other methods are not possible.[9] Methods which do produce effect size estimates are described below; an illustration of their use is provided in Box 16.1.

Box 16.1 Illustration of methods to combine studies

To illustrate the methods for meta-analysis, 17 trials of beta blockers in secondary prevention after myocardial infarction compiled previously are considered.[10] A plot of the effect sizes of these individual studies, together with several pooled estimates, is presented in Figure 16.1. The narrower the 95% confidence intervals, and the larger the plotting symbol, the larger the trial. Clearly trial estimates vary considerably from one another, and although many trials did not attain statistical significance, point estimates exist either side of the line of no treatment effect (odds ratio = 1). This implies there is potentially conflicting information from individual RCTs, and the possibility exists that the treatment is actually harmful. A formal test for heterogeneity is not significant ($\chi^2 = 21 \cdot 7$; $P = 0 \cdot 15$); however the P-value is low enough for concern about heterogeneity, given the low statistical power of the test.

Results from three different models are displayed to illustrate how these affect the pooled estimate. In this instance, the point estimate produced by each method is almost identical. However, this will not always be the case. The fixed effect model produces an estimate which has a narrower confidence interval than the other two methods. The classical and Bayesian (with non-informative priors placed on model parameters) random effects models results are very similar. However, the Bayesian 95% credibility interval is slightly wider than the 95% confidence interval of the classical model. The increase of width observed over the fixed effect model is primarily due to the incorporation of between study heterogeneity. The slight extra inflation of the Bayesian model is due to more parameter uncertainty being taken into account than in the classical random effects model. More recent classical random effects models[11,12] also take this uncertainty into account, and produce similar results to the Bayesian model.

Fixed effect models

A frequently used method to obtain an estimate of overall effect (fixed effect model) takes an average of the primary study estimates, giving a weighting to each which is proportional to its precision. Researchers should report precisely what methods have been used. It should be noted that the fixed effect method assumes all the studies estimate the same, underlying treatment effect, and hence assumes no heterogeneity is present, which may be unrealistic.[13]

SYSTEMATIC REVIEWS OF RANDOMISED TRIALS

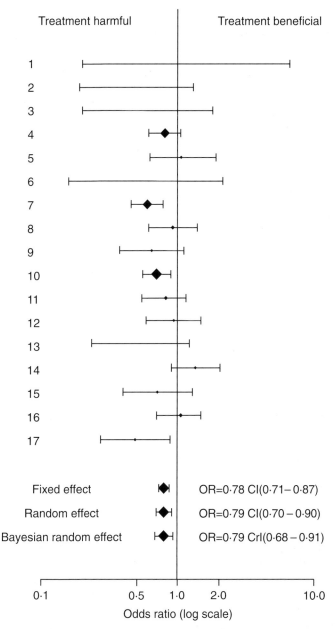

Figure 16.1   Plot of individual effect estimates from beta blocker trials, and pooled results using three different statistical models (fixed effect, random effect, Bayesian random effect).

Random effect models

A model that can incorporate some aspects of heterogeneity when pooling estimates, known as a random effect model,[14] is a popular alternative to the fixed effect method. As a result of incorporating extra variation (that is, accounting for the heterogeneity present between studies), the confidence interval obtained for the pooled estimate is wider than that of the fixed effect method and so is more conservative. The point estimate may also differ, as this method increases the relative weight given to the smaller studies compared to the fixed effect model. Recent work has produced methods that have corrected a previous modelling simplification, and hence incorporate a more appropriate, and usually larger, level of uncertainty for parameters in the model.[11,12] In some instances these approaches produce confidence intervals (for the pooled estimate) which are wider than those of the standard random effects approach. Random effects models have been criticised on grounds that unrealistic or unjustified distributional assumptions have to be made.[15] Neither fixed nor random effect analyses can be considered ideal.[16]

Regression models

Although random effects models allow for heterogeneity between studies, it is desirable, where possible, to explain this variation. This can be achieved by including study level covariates, representing features of the intervention, patients, or study design, which may differ between studies, and may thus explain why estimates of effect differ across studies. When these are included in a fixed effect analysis a meta-regression model results.[17] This idea can be adapted further to produce mixed models, where random effect terms are added to the model. This latter approach may be desirable in instances where covariates explain part of the heterogeneity, but a random effect term is required to accommodate the unexplained remainder.[18] However, such models are used relatively rarely; this is a potentially important approach with which increased experience in practical applications, including criteria for choice of covariates to be included, is needed.

Bayesian methods

As in other areas of health services research, there have been recent developments in the application of Bayesian methods (see Chapter 14).[19] Bayesian methods assume that there may be *a priori* beliefs regarding both the overall intervention effect and the level of between-study heterogeneity. The advantages a Bayesian approach confers include the ability to include pertinent background information that standard classical statistical methods would otherwise exclude, allowing studies to "borrow strength" from one another, and generally allowing for all sources of uncertainty.[20] In addition to these attributes, the Bayesian approach also enables cumulative meta-analyses to be placed within a coherent framework.[21]

Publication and related biases

Publication biases exist because research yielding statistically significant, interesting, or "welcome" results is more likely to be submitted and published (or published quickly).[22] Methods for detecting and/or adjusting for publication bias include: a funnel plot; Rosenthal's file drawer assessment (which estimates how many non-significant studies would have to exist to overturn the pooled result);[23] methods based on weight functions, where the chance of a paper being published is modelled on the significance of its results;[24] and a test recently proposed by Egger.[25] In a similar vein, simulation methods could be adopted to assess the impact of studies which have potentially been missed. Bayesian methods are currently being developed which impute estimated missing studies.[5] Additionally, long-term policy measures, such as registers of all trials commenced, have been suggested as a way of combating this problem.[26] An illustration of implementation of several of these methods is provided in Box 16.2.

Individual patient data

If the original (patient level) data are available from the primary study investigators the option exists of combining and re-analysing the data at the patient level. Advantages of this approach include the ability to carry out detailed data checking, to ensure the appropriateness of the analyses, and to include updated follow-up information.[28] However, such meta-analyses are very time consuming and costly. Currently there is little empirical evidence regarding the actual magnitude of the gains from using patient level data and it is yet to be established whether the extra effort is generally worthwhile, or only in specific situations. Availability of

Box 16.2 Publication bias

A meta-analysis of homoeopathy RCTs[27] illustrates the potential existence of publication bias and the dangers of not accounting for it. A funnel plot (Figure 16.2) of the 89 studies being meta-analysed suggests publication bias may well exist; the left-hand tail is not as large as the right, suggesting the potential omission of small non-significant RCTs. A formal test[25] is statistically significant. It would appear that publication bias is present, which artificially inflates the treatment effect. If the file drawer method is used, assuming all missing RCTs had an average odds ratio of 1 (that is, these trials showed null results on average), it would require 923 missing trials of average size (118 patients) to reduce the pooled effect size to insignificance at the 0·05 level with the random-effects model. When a selection model (based on a weight function)[24] was applied, the pooled odds ratio changed from 2·45 (2·05, 2·93) to 1·78 (1·03, 3·10), a decrease of 27%. However, after this adjustment for publication bias, the result remained highly significant, and since a very large number of unpublished non-significant studies would be needed to overturn this result, it would seem the treatment benefit was not entirely due to publication bias. As an aside the authors comment that in this instance the interpretation of the funnel plot is difficult because they would not expect the effect of homoeopathy to be homogeneous for all clinical conditions, and hence the plot in effect comprises multiple overlapping funnel plots (some centred around no effect, others around real non-zero effects).

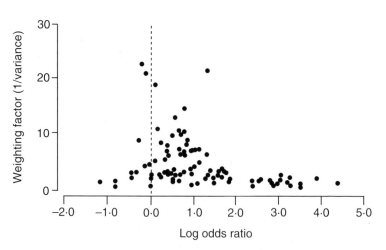

Figure 16.2   Funnel plot of 89 randomised trials included in a meta-analysis.

individual patient data from only a subset of the relevant studies requires development of methods for combining individual patient data together with study level data, including incorporation of both patient-level and study-level covariates.

Generalised synthesis of evidence

In many health care settings evidence is available not only from RCTs but also from non-randomised studies (see Chapters 6 and 7). Methods are being developed for combining evidence from studies of different designs. Cross-design synthesis[29] seeks to capture the strengths of studies and reflect the full range of the available data (from studies of all types). The current methods advocated implement such synthesis using a hierarchical Bayesian modelling approach.[30]

Recommendations

Recommendations for systematic reviews are given below. For the most part these follow standard and widely agreed approaches to these methods.[1,2,4]

- Specification in a protocol of the objectives, hypotheses (in both biological and health care terms), scope, and methods of the systematic review, before the study is undertaken.
- Compilation of as comprehensive a set of reports as possible of relevant primary studies (all potentially relevant data having been searched for), clearly documenting all search methods and sources. Any selection of studies should be based on clearly stated *a priori* specifications.
- Assessment of the methodological quality of each primary study (the method being based on the extent to which susceptibility to bias is minimised – and the specific system used reported). The reproducibility of the procedures in this and the preceding stage should also be assessed.
- Identification of a common set of definitions of outcome, explanatory and confounding variables, that are, as far as possible, compatible with those in each of the primary studies.
- Extraction of estimates of effectiveness and of study and subject characteristics in a standardised way from primary study

documentation, with due checks on extractor bias. Procedures should be explicit, unbiased, and reproducible.

- Where warranted by the scope and characteristics of the data compiled, meta-analysis (quantitative synthesis of primary study results) using appropriate methods and models (clearly stated), in order to explore and allow for all important sources of variation (for example, differences in study quality, participants, in the dose, duration, or nature of the intervention, or in the definitions and measurement of outcomes). Confidence intervals around pooled point estimates should be reported. This will often involve the use of mixed (or hierarchical) models, including fixed covariates to explain some elements of between-study variation, in combination with random effects.

- Where data are too sparse, too low quality, or too heterogeneous to proceed with a statistical aggregation, a narrative or qualitative summary should be performed and the formal meta-analysis omitted. In such cases the process and reporting should still be rigorous and explicit.

- Exploration of the robustness of the results of the systematic review to the choices and assumptions made in all of the above stages. In particular, the following should be explained or explored:
  - the impact of inclusion criteria and study quality;
  - the likelihood and possible impact of publication bias;
  - the implications of the effect of different models and exploration of a reasonable range of values for missing data from studies with uncertain results.

- Clear presentation of key aspects of all of the above stages in the study report, in order to enable critical appraisal and replication of the systematic review. These should include a table of key elements of each primary study. Graphical displays can also assist interpretation and should be included where appropriate.

- Methodological limitations of both the primary studies and the systematic review should be appraised. Any clinical or policy recommendations should be practical and explicit, and make clear the research evidence on which they are based.

References

1. Deeks J, Glanville J, Sheldon T. *Undertaking systematic reviews of research on effectiveness: CRD guidelines for those carrying out or commissioning reviews*, Report no 4. York: CRD, 1996.

2. Oxman AD. *The Cochrane Collaboration handbook: preparing and maintaining systematic reviews.* Oxford: Cochrane Collaboration, 1996.
3. Blair A, Burg J, Foran J *et al.* Guidelines for application of meta-analysis in environmental epidemiology. ISLI Risk Science Institute. *Regul Toxicol Pharmacol* 1995;**22**:189–97.
4. Cook DJ, Sackett DL, Spitzer WO. Methodologic guidelines for systematic reviews of randomized control trials in health care from the Potsdam Consultation on Meta-Analysis. *J Clin Epidemiol* 1995;**48**:167–71.
5. Sutton AJ, Abrams KR, Jones DR, Sheldon TA, Song F. Systematic reviews of trials and other studies. *Health Technol Assess* 1998 (in press).
6. Dickersin K, Scherer R, Lefebvre C. Systematic reviews – identifying relevant studies for systematic reviews. *Br Med J* 1994;**309**:1286–91.
7. Moher D, Klassen TP, Jadad AR, Tugwell P, Moher M, Jones AL. Assessing the quality of randomised controlled trials: implications for the conduct of meta-analyses. *Health Technol Assess* 1998 (in press).
8. Morris RD. Meta-analysis in cancer epidemiology. *Environ Health Perspect* 1994;**102**(Suppl. 8):61–6.
9. Hedges LV, Olkin I. *Statistical methods for meta-analysis.* London: Academic Press, 1985.
10. Egger M, Davey Smith G, Phillips AN. Meta-analysis: principles and procedures. *Br Med J* 1997;**315**:1533–7.
11. Hardy RJ, Thompson SG. A likelihood approach to meta-analysis with random effects. *Statist Med* 1996;**15**:619–29.
12. Biggerstaff BJ, Tweedie RL. Incorporating variability in estimates of heterogeneity in the random effects model in meta-analysis. *Statist Med* 1997;**16**:753–68.
13. Thompson SG, Pocock SJ. Can meta-analyses be trusted? *Lancet* 1991;**338**:1127–30.
14. DerSimonian R, Laird N. Meta-analysis in clinical trials. *Controlled Clin Trials* 1986;**7**:177–88.
15. Peto R. Why do we need systematic overviews of randomised trials? *Statist Med* 1987;**6**:233–40.
16. Thompson SG. Controversies in meta-analysis: the case of the trials of serum cholesterol reduction. *Statist Methods Med Res* 1993;**2**:173–92.
17. Hedges LV. Fixed effects models. In: Cooper H, Hedges LV (eds), *The handbook of research synthesis.* New York: Russell Sage Foundation, 1994.
18. Raudenbush SW. Random effects models. In: Cooper H, Hedges LV (eds), *The handbook of research synthesis.* New York: Russell Sage Foundation, 1994.
19. Spiegelhalter DJ, Myles JP, Jones DR, Abrams KR. Bayesian methods in health technology assessment. *Health Technol Assess* 1998 (in press).
20. Smith TC, Spiegelhalter DJ, Thomas A. Bayesian approaches to random-effects meta-analysis: a comparative study. *Statist Med* 1995;**14**:2685–99.
21. Lau J, Schmid CH, Chalmers TC. Cumulative meta-analysis of clinical trials: builds evidence for exemplary medical care. *J Clin Epidemiol* 1995;**48**:45–57.
22. Easterbrook PJ, Berlin JA, Gopalan R, Matthews DR. Publication bias in clinical research. *Lancet* 1991;**337**:867–72.
23. Rosenthal R. The file drawer problem and tolerance for null results. *Psycholog Bull* 1979;**86**:638–41.
24. Hedges LV. Modeling publication selection effects in meta-analysis. *Statist Sci* 1992;**7**:246–55.
25. Egger M, Smith GD, Schneider M, Minder C. Bias in meta-analysis detected by a simple, graphical test. *Br Med J* 1997;**315**:629–34.
26. Simes RJ. Publication bias: the case for an international registry of clinical trials. *J Clin Oncol* 1986;**4**:1529–41.

27. Linde K, Clausius N, Ramirez G *et al.* Are the clinical effects of homoeopathy placebo effects? A meta-analysis of placebo-controlled trials. *Lancet* 1997;**350**: 834–43.
28. Stewart LA, Clarke MJ. Practical methodology of meta-analyses (overviews) using updated individual patient data. Cochrane Working Group. *Statist Med* 1995;**14**:2057–79.
29. General Accounting Office. *Cross design synthesis: a new strategy for medical effectiveness research.* Washington, DC: General Accounting Office, 1992.
30. Smith TC, Abrams KR, Jones DR. *Using hierarchical models in generalised synthesis of evidence: an example based on studies of breast cancer screening.* Department of Epidemiology and Public Health Technical Report 95-02, University of Leicester, 1995.

17 Handling uncertainty in economic evaluations of health care interventions

ANDREW H BRIGGS AND ALASTAIR M GRAY

The constant introduction of new health technologies, coupled to limited health care resources, has engendered a growing interest in economic evaluation as a way of guiding decision-makers towards interventions likely to offer maximum health gain. In particular, cost-effectiveness analyses – which compare interventions in terms of the extra or incremental cost per unit of health outcome obtained – have become increasingly familiar in many medical and health service journals.

Considerable uncertainty exists when a valid economic evaluation is performed. First, several aspects of the underlying methodological framework are still being debated amongst health economists. Second, there is often considerable uncertainty surrounding the data, the assumptions that may have been used, and how to handle and express this uncertainty. Sensitivity analysis is commonly employed in the absence of patient-level data; however, a number of methods of sensitivity analysis exist with different implications for the interval estimates generated (Box 17.1). Finally, there is a substantial amount of subjectivity in presenting and interpreting the results of economic evaluations.

The aim of this chapter is to give an overview of the handling of uncertainty in economic evaluations of health care interventions.[1] The chapter examines how analysts have handled uncertainty in economic evaluation, assembled data on the distribution and variance of health care costs, and proposed guidelines to improve

Box 17.1 Sensitivity analysis

Sensitivity analysis involves systematically examining the influence of uncertainties in the variables and assumptions employed in an evaluation on the estimated results. It encompasses at least three alternative approaches.[14]

- *One-way sensitivity analysis* systematically examines the impact of each variable in the study by varying it across a plausible range of values while holding all other variables in the analysis constant at their "best-estimate" or baseline value.
- *Extreme scenario analysis* involves setting each variable to simultaneously take the most optimistic (pessimistic) value from the point of view of the intervention under evaluation in order to generate a best (worst) case scenario.

Of course, in real life the components of an evaluation do not vary in isolation nor are they perfectly correlated, hence it is likely that one-way sensitivity analysis will underestimate, and extreme scenario analysis overestimate, the uncertainty associated with the results of economic evaluation.

- A third technique known as *probabilistic sensitivity analysis*, which is based on a large number of Monte Carlo simulations, examines the effect on the results of an evaluation when the underlying variables are allowed to vary simultaneously across a plausible range according to predefined distributions. These probabilistic analyses are likely to produce results that lie between the ranges implied by one-way sensitivity analysis and extreme scenario analysis, and therefore may produce a more realistic estimate of uncertainty.[15]

current practice. It is intended as a contribution towards the development of agreed guidelines for analysts, reviewers, editors, and decision-makers.[2-5]

Nature of the evidence

A structured review examined the methods used to handle uncertainty in the empirical literature, and this was supplemented by a review of methodological articles on the specific topic of confidence interval estimation for cost-effectiveness ratios. The first step in the empirical review was to conduct a search of the literature to identify published economic evaluations that reported results in terms of cost per life year or cost per quality adjusted life year (QALY). This form of study was chosen as it is the results

---

Box 17.2 The "reference case"

The Panel on Cost-Effectiveness in Health and Medicine, an expert committee convened by the US Public Health Service in 1993, proposed that all published cost-effectiveness studies contain at least one set of results based on a standardised set of methods and conventions – a Reference Case analysis – which would aid comparability between studies. The features of this reference case were set out in detail in the panel's report.[3]

The current review used this concept retrospectively, selecting for comparison a subset of results which conformed to the following conditions:

- an incremental analysis was undertaken;
- a health service perspective was employed; and
- both costs and health outcomes were discounted at the UK Treasury approved rate of 6% per annum.

---

of these studies that are commonly considered to be sufficiently comparable to be grouped together and reported in cost-effectiveness league tables.

Searches were conducted for all such studies published up to the end of 1995 using MEDLINE, CINAHL, ECONLIT, Embase, the Social Science Citation Index, and the economic evaluation databases of the Centre for Reviews and Dissemination at York University and the Office of Health Economics/International Federation of Pharmaceutical Manufacturers' Association. Articles identified as meeting the search criteria were reviewed with the use of a form designed to collect summary information on each study, including the disease area, type of intervention, nature of the data, nature of the results, study design, and the methods used to handle uncertainty. This information was entered as keywords into a database to allow interrogation and cross-referencing of the database by category.

This overall dataset was then employed to focus on two specific areas of interest, using subsets of articles to perform more detailed reviews. Firstly, all UK studies were identified and reviewed in detail, and information on the baseline results, the methods underlying those results, the range of results representing uncertainty, and the number of previously published results, quoted for purposes of comparison, were entered onto a relational database. Results were matched by the methods employed with the use of a retrospective application of a methodological "reference case" (Box 17.2);[3] a subset of results with improved comparability was identified and a rank ordering of these results was then attempted. Where a range of values accompanied the baseline results, the implications of this uncertainty for the rank ordering was also examined.

Secondly, all studies that reported patient-level cost data were identified and reviewed in detail with respect to how they had reported the distribution and variance of health care costs. Thirdly, and in parallel with the structured review, five datasets of patient-level cost data were obtained and examined in order to show how the health care costs in those data were distributed and to elucidate issues surrounding the analysis and presentation of health care cost differences.

Economic analyses are not simply concerned with costs, but also with effects, with the incremental cost-effectiveness ratio being the outcome of interest in most economic evaluations. Unfortunately, ratio statistics pose particular problems for standard statistical methods. The review examines a number of proposed methods that have appeared in the recent literature for estimating confidence limits for cost-effectiveness ratios (when patient-level data are available).

Findings

Trends in economic evaluations

A total of 368 articles published up to December 1995 were found to match the search criteria and were fully reviewed. Figure 17.1 shows the studies by year of publication, and indicates an exponential rate of increase. The figure also presents the proportion reporting cost per QALY and cost per life year and shows a trend toward the former. Analysis of the articles in terms of the method employed by analysts to handle uncertainty shows that the vast majority of studies (just over 70%) use one-way sensitivity analysis methods to quantify uncertainty (Box 17.1). Of some concern is that almost 20% of studies did not attempt any analysis to examine uncertainty, although there is weak evidence to show that this situation has improved over time.

Analysis of UK studies

Of the 368 studies, 39 reported results for the UK. From these, 274 baseline results were extracted for different subgroups. The

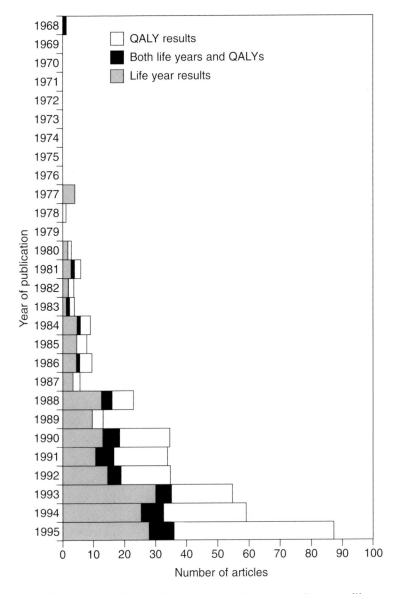

Figure 17.1   Growth in the cost-effectiveness analysis literature reporting cost per life year or cost per QALY.

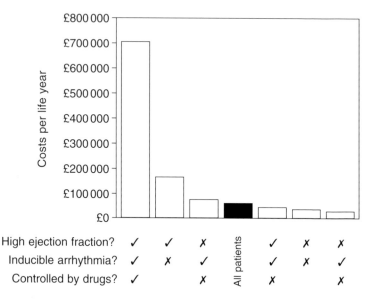

High ejection fraction?	✓	✓	✗	All patients	✓	✗	✗
Inducible arrhythmia?	✓	✗	✓		✓	✗	✓
Controlled by drugs?	✓			✗		✗		✗

Figure 17.2   The importance of sub-group analysis when applying an intervention to patients with different prognostic characteristics: the cost-effectiveness of implantable cardioverter defibrillators.[16]

importance of separate baselines for different subgroups of patients is demonstrated in Figure 17.2, where the average cost per life-year saved of an implantable cardioverter defibrillator (ICD) across the whole patient group – £57 000 – masks important differences between patients with different clinical characteristics. For patients with a low ejection fraction and inducible arrhythmia that is not controlled by drugs, the cost-effectiveness of the ICD device is £22 000 per year of life saved. By contrast, the use of the ICD device in patients with high ejection fraction and inducible arrhythmia that is controlled by drugs is associated with an incremental cost-effectiveness of around £700 000 per year of life saved.

The 274 baseline results used no fewer than 68 different methodological scenarios, and consequently a "reference case" methodological scenario was applied retrospectively to each article; this resulted in a total of 179 methodologically comparable baseline results. These results were converted to a common cost base year and ranked to give a comprehensive "league table" of UK results. Of the 179 results, 50 had an associated range of values to represent uncertainty. Alternative rankings based on the high or low values from this range showed that there could be considerable disruption

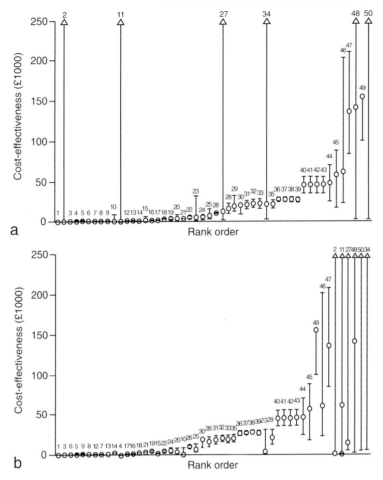

Figure 17.3   Alternative rank orderings of 50 British cost-effectiveness results by (a) baseline value and (b) highest sensitivity analysis value.

to the ranked order based on the baseline point estimates only. This is illustrated by Figure 17.3(a), which shows the rank ordering of these 50 results by their baseline values, and Figure 17.3(b) which shows the same results rank ordered by the highest value from their range. This analysis of UK studies reporting sensitivity analysis ranges raises the further concern that the median number of variables included in the sensitivity analysis was just two. Therefore, the ranges of values shown in Figure 17.3 are likely to be less than if a comprehensive analysis of all uncertain variables had been conducted. Clearly, this would further increase the potential for the rank order to vary depending on the value chosen from the overall range.

Patient-level cost data

Of the 368 studies on the database, only 41 had patient-level cost data and just 20 of these reported some measure of cost variance. Eight reported only range information, which is of limited usefulness in quantifying variance. Only three studies (<1%) had calculated 95% confidence intervals for cost (Figure 17.4).

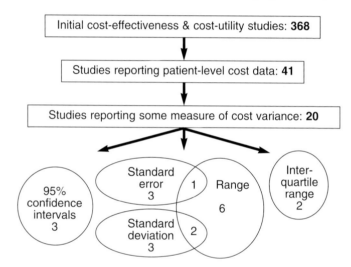

Figure 17.4   The handling of cost variance by studies reporting patient-level cost data.

Turning to the review of the five patient-level cost datasets, analysis indicated that the cost data were not normally distributed. The datasets are presented in Figure 17.5, with an overlay showing the normal distribution of same mean and variance. The figure clearly shows that many cost data are substantially skewed in their distribution. This may cause problems for parametric statistical tests for the equality of two means. One method for dealing with this is to transform the data to an alternative scale of measurement, for example by means of log, square root, or reciprocal transformations. However, our analysis of these data indicated that while a transformation may modestly improve the statistical

194

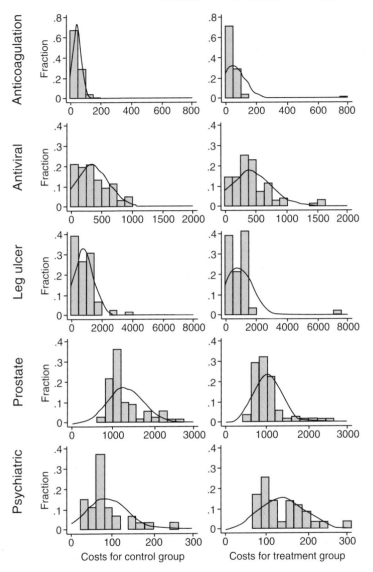

Figure 17.5 Distributions of cost in the control and treatment arms of five datasets reporting patient-level cost data.

significance of observed cost differences, or reduce the sample size requirements to detect a specified difference, it is very difficult to give the results of a transformed or back transformed scale a

195

meaningful economic interpretation, especially if we intend to use the cost information as part of a cost-effectiveness ratio. It would be appropriate to use non-parametric bootstrapping to test whether the sample size of a study's cost data is sufficient for the central limit theorem to hold, and wherever possible to base analyses on mean values from untransformed data.

Estimating confidence intervals for cost-effectiveness ratios

Finally, our review identified a number of different methods for estimating confidence intervals for cost-effectiveness ratios that have appeared in the recent literature,[6-11] and applied each of these methods to one of the five datasets listed above.[12] These different methods can produce very different intervals as shown in Figure 17.6. Examination of their statistical properties and evidence from recent Monte Carlo simulation studies[11,13] suggests that many of these methods may not perform well in some circumstances. The parametric method based on Fieller's theorem and the non-parametric approach of bootstrapping have been shown to produce consistently the best results in terms of the number of times, in repeated sampling, the true population parameter is contained within the interval.[11,13]

Recommendations

Uncertainty in economic evaluation is often handled inconsistently and unsatisfactorily. Recently published guidelines should improve this situation, but we would emphasise the following:

- ensure that the potential implications of uncertainty for the results are considered in all analyses;
- when reporting cost and cost-effectiveness information, make more use of descriptive statistics. Interval estimates should accompany each point estimate presented;
- sensitivity analyses should be comprehensive in their inclusion of all variables;
- cost and cost-effectiveness data are often skewed. Significance tests may be more powerful on a transformed scale, but confidence limits should be reported on the original scale. Even

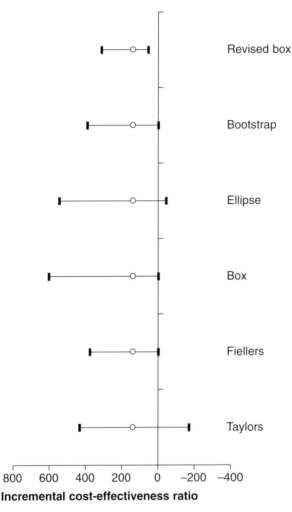

Figure 17.6 Confidence intervals for cost-effectiveness ratios using different methods proposed in the recent literature.

when data are skewed, economic analyses should, where possible, be based on means of distributions;

• where patient-level data on both cost and effect are available, the parametric approach based on Fieller's theorem or the non-parametric approach of bootstrapping should be employed to estimate a confidence interval for the cost-effectiveness ratio;

- when comparing results between studies, ensure the comparators are representative; and
- using a methodological reference case when presenting results will increase the comparability of results between studies.

References

1. Briggs AH, Gray AM. Handling uncertainty when performing economic evaluations of health care interventions: a systematic review with special reference to the variance and distributional form of cost data. *Health Technol Assess* (in press).
2. Drummond MF, Jefferson TO. Guidelines for authors and peer reviewers of economic submissions to the BMJ. *Br Med J* 1996;**313**:275–83.
3. Gold MR, Siegel JE, Russell LB *et al. Cost-effectiveness in health and medicine.* Oxford: Oxford University Press, 1996.
4. Canadian Coordinating Office for Health Technology Assessment. *Guidelines for the economic evaluation of pharmaceuticals.* Ottawa: Canadian Coordinating Office for Health Technology Assessment (CCOHTA), 2nd edn, 1997.
5. Drummond MF, O'Brien B, Stoddart GL *et al. Methods for the economic evaluation of health care programmes* Oxford: Oxford University Press, 2nd edn., 1997.
6. O'Brien BJ, Drummond MF, Labelle RJ, Willan A. In search of power and significance: issues in the design and analysis of stochastic cost-effectiveness studies in health care. *Med Care* 1994;**32**:150–63.
7. Wakker P, Klaassen M. Confidence intervals for cost-effectiveness ratios. *Health Economics* 1995;**4**:373–82.
8. van Hout BA, Al MJ, Gordon GS, Rutten FF. Costs, effects and C/E-ratios alongside a clinical trial. *Health Economics* 1994;**3**:309–19.
9. Chaudhary MA, Stearns SC. Estimating confidence intervals for cost-effectiveness ratios: an example from a randomised trial. *Statist Med* 1996;**15**: 1447–58.
10. Briggs AH, Wonderling DE, Mooney CZ. Pulling cost-effectiveness analysis up by its bootstraps: a non-parametric approach to confidence interval estimation. *Health Economics* 1997;**6**:327–40.
11. Polsky D, Glick HA, Willke R, Schulman K. Confidence intervals for cost-effectiveness ratios: a comparison of four methods. *Health Economics* 1997;**6**: 243–52.
12. Fenn P, McGuire A, Phillips V, Backhouse M, Jones D. The analysis of censored treatment cost data in economic evaluation. *Med Care* 1995;**33**: 851–63.
13. Briggs AH, Mooney CZ, Wonderling DE. Constructing confidence intervals around cost-effectiveness ratios: an evaluation of parametric and non-parametric methods using Monte Carlo simulation. *Statist Med* (in press).
14. Briggs AH. *Handling uncertainty in the results of economic evaluation.* OHE Briefing Paper No.32, 1995.
15. Manning WG, Fryback DG, Weinstein MC. Reflecting uncertainty in cost-effectiveness analysis. In: Gold MR, Siegel JE, Russell LB, Weinstein MC (eds). *Cost-effectiveness in health and medicine.* Oxford: Oxford University Press, 1996.
16. Anderson MH, Camm AJ. Implications for present and future applications of the implantable cardioverter-defibrillator resulting from the use of a simple model of cost efficacy. *Br Heart J* 1993;**69**:83–92.

18 Consensus development methods for creating clinical guidelines

NICK BLACK, MAGGIE MURPHY,
DONNA LAMPING, MARTIN McKEE,
COLIN SANDERSON, JANET ASKHAM
AND THERESA MARTEAU

Clinicians, managers, and policy-makers regularly make difficult choices. In an ideal world, such decisions would be based on evidence derived from rigorously conducted empirical studies. In practice, there are many areas of health care where insufficient research evidence exists, or may never exist.[1] Informed decisions, in such circumstances, have of necessity to be based partly on the opinions of those with personal knowledge and experience of the subject.[2] To help, a variety of formal consensus development methods have been devised for capturing informed judgements given incomplete research evidence and the need to resolve differences of opinion.

The most common use of consensus development methods in health services has been in the creation of clinical guidelines. Although there is debate about the appropriate place of guidelines in clinical practice, they are recognised as one way of assisting clinicians in decision-making. This chapter reviews the methodological factors that can shape and influence clinical guidelines created through consensus development, and makes recommendations about best practice in the use of such methods.

199

Nature of the evidence

This review is restricted to a consideration of formal consensus development methods in which the inputs, processes, and the nature of the desired outputs are made explicit to the participants before the start. Such formal methods generally have advantages over informal ones in which groups make decisions without any

---

Box 18.1 Assumptions about decision-making in groups and the advantages of formal methods

- *Safety in numbers* – several people are less likely to arrive at a wrong decision than a single individual
- *Authority* – a selected group of individuals is more likely to lend some authority to the decision produced
- *Rationality* – decisions are improved by reasoned argument in which assumptions are challenged and members forced to justify their views
- *Controlled process* – by providing a structured process, formal methods can eliminate negative aspects of group decision-making
- *Scientific credibility* – formal consensus development methods meet the requirements of scientific methods

---

pre-arranged rules (Box 18.1).[3,4] The majority of the literature reviewed was identified through searches of electronic bibliographic databases (MEDLINE, PsychLIT, SSCI) and through the reference lists of retrieved articles. In all, 177 primary research and review articles were selected.[5]

It should also be recognised that the principal constraint in assessing the research evidence is the problem of assessing the validity of many consensus decisions because of the absence of an objective "gold standard".

A considerable amount of research has been carried out on consensus development methods but many aspects remain under- or uninvestigated. For the time being at least, advice on those aspects has, therefore, to be based on the experience of those who have used or participated in these methods plus users' commonsense. To avoid confusion, the extent to which research support exists for any finding is indicated:

[A] = clear research evidence;
[B] = limited supporting research evidence;
[C] = experienced or commonsense judgement.

These should not necessarily be considered as a hierarchy, as some aspects of consensus development methods are either not amenable to or inappropriate for scientific study.

Findings

Three main approaches have been used in health services. In the 1950s the Delphi method was introduced;[6] this was followed by the nominal group technique (NGT) in the 1960s;[7] and in 1977, the consensus development conference.[8] The main features of these methods, along with some other methods, are shown in Table 18.1. The most frequently used method for clinical guideline development is the NGT, as this permits consideration of a large number of detailed clinical situations (scenarios). NGTs will be the main focus of this chapter. The other methods have been more widely used for forecasting, prioritisation, and broad policy development.

Although the NGT can take a variety of forms, it has several key features. First, each participant records his or her ideas independently and privately. Commonly the ideas are then listed in a round-robin format, that is one idea is collected from each individual in turn and listed by a group facilitator, continuing until all ideas have been listed. The ideas are then discussed in turn by the group before the participants privately rate their strength of support for each idea. The individual judgements are aggregated statistically to derive the group judgement. The principal features of one of the most frequently used forms of NGT are shown in Box 18.2.

While the planning and conduct of consensus development are to some extent based on an iterative process, a review of the research evidence is best based on the following sequence of decisions and events:

- setting the task/s or question/s to be addressed;
- selecting the participants;
- choosing and preparing the scientific evidence to provide for participants;
- structuring the interaction; and
- synthesising the participants' individual judgements.

Table 18.1 Characteristics of informal and formal consensus development methods

	Mailed questionnaires	Private decisions elicited	Formal feedback of group choices	Face-to-face contact	Interaction structured	Aggregation method
Informal	No	No	No	Yes	No	Implicit
Delphi method	Yes	Yes	Yes	No	Yes	Explicit
NGT	No	Yes	Yes	Yes	Yes	Explicit
RAND version	Yes	Yes	Yes	Yes	Yes	Explicit
Consensus development conference	No	No	No	Yes	No*	Implicit
Other methods						
Staticised group	No	Yes	No	No	–	Explicit
Social judgement analysis	No	Yes	Yes	Yes	No	Implicit
Structured discussion	No	No	No	Yes	Yes	Implicit

* Although there may be no pre-arranged structure to the group interaction, groups may adopt formal rules.

Box 18.2 The RAND form of a nominal group technique

A nine-member group of experts first defines a set of indications to reflect its concepts of the critical factors (or cues) in decision-making for patients with the condition. The participants are chosen because of their clinical expertise, influence, and geographic location. Furthermore, they may represent academic and community practice and different specialties.

After agreeing on definitions and the structure of the indications (scenarios), the participants rate the indications using a 9-point scale where 1 = extremely inappropriate (risks greatly exceed benefits), 5 = uncertain (benefits and risks about equal), and 9 = extremely appropriate (benefits greatly exceed risks). By appropriate, it is meant that the expected health benefits to an average patient exceed the expected health risks by a sufficiently wide margin that the intervention is worthwhile and it is superior to alternatives (including no intervention).

The final ratings of appropriateness are the result of a two-stage process. The indications are initially rated independently by each participant without discussion or contact with the others. The group then assemble and the collated ratings are presented for discussion. After discussion, each participant independently and confidentially rerates each indication. The median rating is used as the appropriateness score.

To determine agreement and disagreement a statistical definition using the binomial distribution is applied. For a nine-member group, agreement exists when no more than two individuals rate a particular indication outside a 3-point range (that is 1–3, 4–6, 7–9). Disagreement about an indication exists when three or more rate a particular indication 7–9 and another three rate the same indication in the 1–3 range. Other indications are regarded either as equivocal (agreement at the centre of the scale) or as partial agreement.

(Based on Bernstein et al.)[9]

Setting the task/s or question/s to be addressed

Considerable care must be given to the selection of the cues – the characteristics that influence clinical management, such as the severity of the patient's condition (Box 18.3). Participants should be given the opportunity to say which cues they consider important as doing so may help maintain their participation and help them justify their judgements. Participants' views of the relevant cues can usefully be obtained during a preliminary round of individual open-ended consultations. [C]

Box 18.3 Setting the task/s or question/s to be addressed for determining the appropriate indications for cholecystectomy

- *Cues to be considered*
  - medical history (severity and nature of pain; length of history; jaundice)
  - pathological findings (number and size of stones in gall bladder; stones in common bile duct; gall bladder functioning or not; common bile duct dilated or not)
  - comorbid conditions (none; mild; moderate; severe)
- *Scenarios to be included*
  - limited to those which occur at least once a year in a typical surgeon's work
- *Contextual cues*
  - assume reality of resource availability in the existing health care system
- *Other relevant interventions*
  - assume endoscopic sphincterotomy has not yet been attempted so this alternative is available
- *Type of judgement*
  - overall judgement as to whether or not surgery is appropriate in each scenario considered

---

Contextual cues (such as whether judgements should assume unlimited health care resources or the reality of restricted resources) are as important as those specific to the topic. Participants are likely to make differing assumptions about these cues if they are not specified in the task, so it is important to make them explicit.[10] **[B]**

The focus of the task may either be ways of managing a particular condition or the indications for using an intervention. If the latter, care needs to be taken as to how other relevant interventions are dealt with because views of the appropriateness of any intervention will depend on whether or not the possibility of using alternative interventions is taken into account. Ambiguity as to whether or not alternatives should be considered can affect group consensus. For example, participants may be instructed either to make their judgements in terms of the intervention under consideration being more or less appropriate than other interventions in general or than some specified intervention/s. **[C]**

Participants may be asked to provide an overall judgement (for example, treatment is or is not appropriate in a particular scenario) or an attempt can be made to break the judgement down into probability and utility estimates.[11] There are theoretical advantages with the latter but it is likely to be a more difficult task for some participants (probability estimates are a matter for technical experts, though utility estimates may appropriately involve others, including patients) and it is unclear whether it enhances judgements. [C]

Although including all theoretically possible scenarios will increase the comprehensiveness of the exercise, if many of the scenarios rarely occur in practice, the increased burden on the participants may not be justified by the limited value of the information provided.[12] It is also likely that judgements of scenarios which never or rarely occur are less reliable than judgements of scenarios which more commonly occur in practice. [B] Further, requiring participants to judge what may be seen as numerous irrelevant scenarios may alienate them from the task. [C]

Selecting the participants

Within defined specialist or professional categories, the selection of the particular individuals is likely to have little impact on the group decision as long as the group is of sufficient size.[1,13] To enhance the credibility and widespread acceptance of the guidelines, it is advisable that the participants reflect the full range of key characteristics of the population they are intended to influence. The basis for selection should also be seen to be unbiased. [C]

Whether a homogeneous or heterogeneous group, defined in terms of specialist or professional characteristics, is best will in part depend on the purpose of the exercise.[14] If the aim is to define common ground and maximise areas of agreement, groups should be homogeneous in composition. If, in contrast, the aim is to identify and explore areas of uncertainty, a heterogeneous group is appropriate. [B]

In judgements of clinical appropriateness, the most influential characteristic of participants is their medical specialty. Specialists tend to favour the interventions they are most familiar with (Table 18.2).[15–17] Consensus-based guidelines should therefore be interpreted in the context of the specialty composition of the group. [A]

In general, having more group members will increase the reliability of group judgement (Figure 18.1).[18] However, large

205

Table 18.2 Comparison of proportion of indications judged to be appropriate according to specialist and to mixed groups

Topic	Specialist group (%)	Mixed group (%)
Cholecystectomy[15]		
Agreement	61	67
appropriate	29	13
equivocal	5	4
inappropriate	27	50
Partial agreement	31	18
Disagreement	8	15
Carotid endarterectomy[16]		
appropriate	70	38
equivocal	10	31
inappropriate	19	31
Spinal manipulation[17]		
appropriate	33	9
uncertain	22	37
inappropriate	45	54

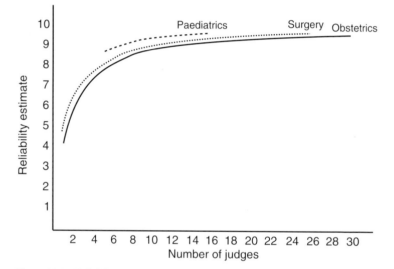

Figure 18.1 Reliability of group decision according to number of judges in three medical specialties.

groups may cause coordination problems. Although it is theoretically likely that group size will affect decision-making, the effects are subtle and difficult to detect.[19] Below about six participants, reliability will decline quite rapidly, while above about 12, improvements in reliability will be subject to diminishing returns. [**B**]

Choosing and preparing the scientific evidence

Such research-based information as is available should be provided to all participants at an early stage because:

- if all members of the group have access to such information, it is more likely to be discussed within the group;
- providing a literature review to group members before discussion may enhance the perception that the task is research-based, which will in turn encourage members to be more reliant on information; and
- providing a common starting point may foster group cohesion. [C]

Participants should be encouraged to bring the review and any personal notes to the group sessions as a memory aid. Information presented in the form of articles or abstracts is less easily assimilated than information presented in a synthesised form, such as tables.[20] Presenting information in an easy to read and understandable format may mean participants are more likely to use it. Tabulating the information in a way which increases the salience of the cues to be used for making judgements means that the information is more likely to be processed in this manner.[21] [C]

Those with expertise in judging the quality of scientific research should be involved in conducting any literature review. Organisation of materials by methodologists can highlight those factors which are most relevant to making a judgement, thus making it more likely that judgements will be based on the appropriate information. [C] Grading the quality of studies with a reliable method (such as a standard checklist) may mitigate the biases of the reviewers somewhat, but may not eliminate them. [B]

Structuring the interaction

Two or three rating rounds are likely to result in some convergence of individual judgements (Table 18.3). [A] More than three rounds is likely to have little impact on the level of agreement and to have adverse effects on the response rate. [C]

The status of participants is known to affect their contribution to and influence within a group so efforts should be made to mitigate this (for example, by the use of confidential methods for participants to record their views). [B]

Table 18.3 Change in mean deviation from the median for initial and final ratings using a NGT

		Initial rating	Final rating	Amount of change
Park et al.	Coronary angiography	1·37	0·86	−0·52
(1986)[23]	CABG	1·58	1·06	−0·64
	Cholecystectomy	1·29	0·98	−0·31
	Endoscopy	1·39	0·83	−0·56
	Colonoscopy	1·91	1·36	−0·55
	Carotid endarterectomy	0·52	0·34	−0·17
Scott & Black	Cholecystectomy			
(1991)[22]	mixed group	1·25	0·95	−0·30
	surgical group	1·16	1·02	−0·14
Matcher et al.	Carotid endarterectomy	1·24	0·95	−0·29
(1992)[24]				
Bernstein et al.	Coronary angiography	1·53	1·22	−0·31
(1992)[9]				
Ballard et al.	Abdominal aortic			
(1992)[25]	aneurysm surgery	1·10	1·00	−0·10
Coulter et al.	Spinal manipulation			
(1995)[17]	mixed group	1·70	1·14	−0·54
	chiropractic group	1·39	0·83	−0·56

If a NGT is being used, a comfortable environment for meetings is likely to be preferred by participants and to be conducive to discussion.[26] In addition, a good facilitator will enhance consensus development and can ensure that the procedure is conducted according to agreed procedures.[27] [C]

Methods of synthesising individual judgements

An implicit approach to aggregating individual judgements may be adequate for establishing broad policy guidelines but more explicit methods based on quantitative analysis are needed to develop detailed, clinical guidelines. [C]

The level of agreement within a group is more dependent on whether or not outliers (individuals with extreme views) are included, than on how agreement is defined (for example "all individual ratings identical" versus "all within a three-point range") (Table 18.4). The exclusion of outliers can have a marked effect on the content of guidelines.[12,22,29] [A] If the definition of agreement is too demanding (such as requiring all individuals' ratings to be

Table 18.4   Impact of different definitions of agreement on the proportion of scenarios about which the group reached agreement

	Include all ratings		Exclude furthest ratings		Exclude min–max ratings	
	Strict	Relaxed	Strict	Relaxed	Strict	Relaxed
Park et al. (1989)[12]						
Coronary angiography	28·0	28·7	–	–	50·0	56·3
Endoscopy	25·4	25·4	–	–	41·3	41·6
Carotid endarterectomy	40·9	40·9	–	–	53·4	53·8
Scott & Black (1991)[22]						
Cholecystectomy						
mixed panel	45·0	47·0	63·0	67·0	–	–
surgical panel	35·0	35·0	57·0	61·0	50·0	53·0
Imamura et al. (1997)[28]						
Total hip replacement						
Britain	41·5	41·5	52·8	59·4	48·1	51·9
Japan	23·3	31·7	50·0	68·9	44·2	55·0

Strict = all ratings in one of three predefined ranges 1–3, 4–6, 7–9
Relaxed = all ratings within any 3-point range

identical) either no statements will qualify or those that do will be of little interest. [C]

Differential weighting of individual participants' views can only be justified if there is a clear empirical basis, related to the task, for calculating the weights. There is no agreement as to the best method of mathematical aggregation.[30] [B] An indication of the distribution or dispersal of participants' judgements should be reported and not just the measure of central tendency. In general, the median and the interquartile range are more robust to the influence of outliers than the mean and standard deviation. [A]

Recommendations

Like all methods, NGTs and other consensus development methods have their shortcomings. This is not a reason for rejecting them but, as with any scientific method, this should serve to remind users to remain aware of the likely effects that various methodological features may have on the results. Similarly, recipients of clinical guidelines developed using these methods should interpret them in the light of how the method was applied. For example, how homogeneous was the composition of the group and what were the members' backgrounds? A full checklist, based on this review of the literature, for judging the process of developing particular consensus-based guidelines is being prepared.

References

1. Chassin M. How do we decide whether an investigation or procedure is appropriate? In: Hopkins A (ed.), *Appropriate investigation and treatment in clinical practice*. London: Royal College of Physicians, 1989.
2. Agency for Health Care and Policy Research. *Clinical Practice Guideline Program. Report to Congress.* Rockville, Maryland: AHCPR, US Department of Health and Human Services, 1995.
3. Asch SE. Studies of independence and conformity: a minority of one against a unanimous majority. *Psycholog Monographs* 1956;70(9):No.416.
4. Janis I. *Groupthink* Boston: Houghton-Mifflin, 2nd edn. 1982.
5. Murphy M, Black NA, Lamping D *et al.* Consensus development methods, and their use in clinical guideline development. *Health Technol Assess* 1998; 2(3):1–88.
6. Dalkey NC, Helmer O. An experimental application of the Delphi method to the use of experts. *Manag Sci* 1963;9:458–67.
7. Delbecq A, van de Ven A. A group process model for problem identification and program planning. *J Appl Behav Sci* 1971;7:467–92.
8. Fink A, Kosecoff J, Chassin M, Brook RH. Consensus methods: characteristics and guidelines for use. *Am J Public Health* 1984;74:979–83.
9. Bernstein SJ, Laouri M, Hilborne LH *et al. Coronary angiography: a literature review and ratings of appropriateness and necessity.* Report JRA-03. Santa Monica, CA: RAND, 1992.
10. Brook RH, Kosecoff JB, Park RE, Chassin MR, Winslow CM, Hampton JR. Diagnosis and treatment of coronary disease: comparison of doctors' attitudes in the USA and the UK. *Lancet* 1988;i:750–3.
11. Silverstein MD, Ballard DJ. Expert panel assessment of appropriateness of abdominal aortic aneurysm surgery: global judgement versus probability estimates. *J Health Serv Res Policy* 1998;3:134–40.
12. Park RE, Fink A, Brook RH *et al.* Physician ratings of appropriate indications for three procedures: theoretical indications vs indications used in practice. *Am J Public Health* 1989;79:445–7.
13. Kastein MR, Jacobs M, van der Hell RH, Luttik K, Touw-Otten FWMM. Delphi, the issue of reliability: a qualitative Delphi study in primary health care in the Netherlands. *Technol Forecasting Social Change* 1993;44:315–23.
14. Jehn KA. A multimethod examination of the benefits and detriments of intragroup conflict. *Admin Sci Quart* 1995;40:256–82.
15. Scott EA, Black NA. When does consensus exist in expert panels? *J Public Health Med* 1991;13:35–9.
16. Leape LL, Park RE, Kahan JP, Brook RH. Group judgments of appropriateness: the effect of panel composition. *Quality Assurance Health Care* 1992;4:151–9.
17. Coulter I, Adams A, Shekelle P. Impact of varying panel membership on ratings of appropriateness in consensus panels: a comparison of a multi- and single disciplinary panel. *Health Services Res* 1995;30:577–91.
18. Richardson FM. Peer review of medical care. *Med Care* 1972;10:29–39.
19. Davis JH. Some compelling intuitions about group consensus decisions, theoretical and empirical research, and interpersonal aggregation phenomena: selected examples, 1950–1990. *Organiz Behav Human Decision Processes* 1992; 52:3–38.
20. Payne JW, Bettman JR, Johnson EJ. Behavioral decision research: a constructive processing perspective. *Ann Rev Psychol* 1992;43:87–131.
21. Bettman JR, Kakkar P. Effects of information presentation format on consumer information acquisition strategies. *J Consumer Res* 1977;3:233–40.

22. Scott EA, Black NA. Appropriateness of cholecystectomy in the United Kingdom – a consensus panel approach. *Gut* 1991;**32**:1066–70.
23. Park RE, Fink A, Brook RH *et al*. Physician ratings of appropriate indications for six medical and surgical procedures. R-3280-CWF/HF/PMT/RJW. Santa Monica, CA: RAND, 1986.
24. Matcher DB, Goldstein LB, McCrory DC *et al*. Carotid endarterectomy: a literature review and ratings of appropriateness and necessity. Report JRA-05. Santa Monica, CA: RAND, 1992.
25. Ballard DJ, Etchason JA, Hilbourne LH *et al*. Abdominal aortic aneurysm surgery: a literature review and ratings of appropriateness and necessity. Report JRA-04. Santa Monica, CA: RAND, 1992.
26. Reagan-Cirincione P, Rohrbaugh J. Decision conferencing: a unique approach to the behavioral aggregation of expert judgment. In: Wright G, Bolger F. *Expertise and decision support*, New York: Plenum Press, 1992.
27. Vinokur A, Burnstein E, Sechrest L, Wortman PM. Group decision making by experts: field study of panels evaluating medical technologies. *J Personal Social Psychol* 1985;**49**:70–84.
28. Imamura K, Gair R, McKee M, Black N. Appropriateness of total hip replacement in the United Kingdom. *World Hospitals Health Services* 1997;**32**: 10–14.
29. Naylor CD, Basinski A, Baigrie RS, Goldman BS, Lomas J. Placing patients in the queue for coronary revascularization: evidence for practice variations from an expert panel process. *Am J Public Health* 1990; **80**:1246–52.
30. Kozlowski SWJ, Hattrup K. A disagreement about within-group agreement: disentangling issues of consistency versus consensus. *J Appl Psychol* 1992;**77**: 161–7.

Part Five
Future developments

19 Horizon scanning: early identification of new health care technologies

GLENN ROBERT, ANDREW STEVENS AND JOHN GABBAY

The introduction of new health care technologies (whether drugs, devices, procedures, or innovative ways of delivering services) can have enormous consequences, both desirable and undesirable, for health services and patients. New technologies are often introduced in a haphazard and uncontrolled manner causing unnecessary confusion or expense.[1,2]

Around 100 new drugs (including major new indications) are introduced each year with increasing policy and expenditure implications. For example, beta interferon for multiple sclerosis could cost £400 million a year in the United Kingdom, yet many questions have been raised about its usefulness and we continue to await a randomised trial with generalisable findings which allows an accurate assessment of cost and benefit. Research-based evidence on cost-effectiveness (not just safety and efficacy) is the only way to establish the appropriate use of any technology.[3] Earlier identification of beta interferon as a new technology could have helped to ensure research evidence was available prior to its marketing and introduction.[4] The introduction of other types of health care technologies that have had large implications has also been uncontrolled; the uptake of laparoscopic surgery in the early 1990s has been termed the "biggest unaudited free-for-all in the history of surgery".[5]

Since the 1970s, studies of biomedical innovation and of the diffusion of health care technology have become more frequent, and slowly knowledge is accumulating about the complex process of their development and use (Figure 19.1).[6] Most discussions

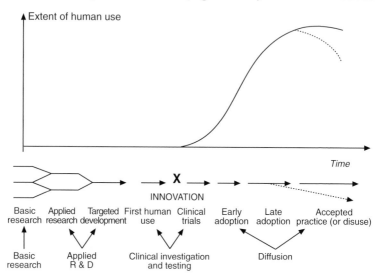

Figure 19.1   Stages in the development and diffusion of health care technologies (Office of Technology Assessment, USA).

share the conclusion that diffusion is a process best represented by an S-shaped curve[7] in which adoption is gradual at first, picks up speed as positive experience reduces both uncertainty and ignorance about the innovation, and finally slows down as fewer individuals remain who do not use it. However, the development of an innovation is unpredictable and can be complex;[8] for example, progress in five different biomedical research programmes (X-ray, tomographic techniques, instrumentation, mathematics, and computers) were required in order to develop computed tomography scanners.[9] Furthermore, many innovations will never be introduced to clinical practice at all; the attrition rate of pharmaceuticals in the second half of the 1970s was such that of roughly every 10 000 compounds synthesised, 1000 underwent animal testing, 10 were selected for human testing, and ultimately only one made it to the health care market.[10] Similarly, only a small number of the potential new products for which patents have been issued will ultimately be introduced into clinical practice.[11]

Even in the early adoption stage many uncertainties remain, often concerning the precise indications and/or patients for which the technology will eventually be used. In addition, the cost and effectiveness of new innovations often remain uncertain long after their initial adoption. These factors mean that forecasts have to be largely subjective and that it is necessary to undertake assessments of cost-effectiveness "early and often".[12] Clearly, early identification of impending technologies can help in this regard and can also help to fulfil a number of other objectives (Box 19.1).[13] This

---

Box 19.1 Objectives of early warning of impending technologies

- To develop and prioritise a health technology assessment programme
- To assist with issuing guidance to health service purchasers and providers about the use of new advances
- To estimate future cost implications
- To consider the implications for planning the configuration of health services
- To encourage professional bodies to develop any necessary guidance and to assess implications for standards and training

---

chapter considers which sources should be used to provide such intelligence and considers how an early warning system might operate.

Nature of the evidence

A review of studies predicting future aspects of health care (Box 19.2) was carried out, together with a telephone survey of coordinators of existing and planned early warning systems from around the world and an international Delphi survey (see Chapter 18). In addition, we undertook nine retrospective case studies to obtain lessons on how specific innovations could have been identified prior to their introduction to health services. The aim of the telephone survey was to ascertain how other countries' early warning systems were organised. Semistructured questionnaires to six respondents focused on the aims, methods, and level of support of each of the early warning systems. In the Delphi survey we used 38 participants and three rounds to devise and develop a

---

Box 19.2 Three types of literature related to future aspects of health care

Several studies have used formal and empirical methods to identify health care technologies likely to be introduced to a health care system within a short time-span; a few went further and provided a critique of the various sources of information and methods which might be adopted for the purposes of an early warning system.[11,14-17]

In addition, there are vast numbers of discursive papers, often editorials, about future developments in particular areas of health care. These are unsystematic and mostly written from one person's perspective. In many cases, the judgements are made by experts who have personal enthusiasms and an "insider" perspective.[18] Relying on such sources might not detect all emerging health care technologies nor correctly assess their potential.

Numerous papers describe the application of futures techniques (such as Delphi surveys and scenario analyses) to health care. However, these often take a very broad and long-term approach, examining demographic and scientific trends, as opposed to identifying specific imminent technologies and were therefore not considered further.

---

classification of health care technologies, and to assess potential sources for identifying each type.

Given the lack of empirical evidence with which to assess the validity of the results of the Delphi survey, we carried out nine retrospective case studies to assess whether the recommended sources would have been able to identify important health care technologies *prior* to their launch or initial adoption. The case studies, chosen to give a range of different types, were: beta interferon for multiple sclerosis; dornase alfa for cystic fibrosis; donepezil for Alzheimer's disease; the Medisense ExacTech pen (a biosensor); left ventricular assist devices as a bridge to heart transplantation; telemedicine; computed tomography scanners; paediatric intensive care units; and laparoscopic cholecystectomy.

Findings

Existing initiatives

There exists no agreed or empirically proven method of identifying and predicting the likely future impact of new health care

218

technologies. However, six national organisations are currently attempting to establish such systems. These aim not only to establish research priorities for health technology assessment but to inform professional groups and other interested parties. Their activities can provide clinicians with early warning to allow time for the preparation of guidelines, or to inform decisions as to when expenditure on a new advance is justified or not. Often there are existing schemes and programmes that can helpfully contribute to an overall early warning system in any country but they need to be coordinated and supplemented by additional sources of information (for example, pharmacist networks may collaborate to provide advance information on significant new drugs in development).[19]

The most striking aspect of the national initiatives is, with the exception of The Netherlands,[11,16-17] how recently they have been established (Table 19.1). Many other health futures initiatives have

Table 19.1   National early warning initiatives

Country	Date began	Organisation
The Netherlands	1988	Health Council of The Netherlands
United Kingdom	1995	NHS R&D HTA Programme[20]
Canada	1997	Canadian Co-ordinating Office for Health Technology Assessment
France	1997	Agence Nationale d'Accreditation et d'Evaluation en Santé
Sweden	1998	Swedish Council on Technology Assessment in Health Care
Denmark	planned 1998	Danish Institute for Technology Assessment in Health Care

either been broad and long-ranging, looking at the future in terms of societal, technical, and demographic change,[21] or used *ad hoc* expert panels to consider a particular disease or specialty.[22] However, few of these have clearly identified technologies which have a major impact in the short term on the outcome and cost of providing health care.

Information sources

The information sources that countries have adopted and further sources which were identified in the Delphi survey are shown in

---

Box 19.3 Categorisation of potential sources of information for "horizon scanning"

- Primary
  - Patents
  - Early pharmaceutical trial registration
  - Pharmaceutical, biotechnology, and medical engineering companies
- Secondary
  - Published literature (scientific, pharmaceutical, medical) using scanning and focused searching
  - Expert opinion by way of either written surveys either focused or general or in-depth interviews
  - Conferences
  - News services; including the financial press
  - Financial markets
  - Specialist registers (e.g. Safety & Efficacy Register of New Interventional Procedures)
  - Licensing applications
  - Research funding sources
  - Regulatory organisations (e.g. European Union; US Food and Drug Administration)
  - Private health care providers
  - Patient special interest groups
- Tertiary
  - Health technology assessment newsletters; links with other agencies; other early warning systems

---

Box 19.3. Primary information sources (manufacturer/innovator information) are likely to provide earlier warning but are uncertain indicators of when the technology will be adopted, if ever. For example, patents were issued for a computed tomography scanner in 1961 and 1962 but it was not until the early 1970s that the technology entered clinical use. Primary sources often provide little detail on the potential new technology. *Secondary* (knowledge or expertise intended for other purposes) and *tertiary* (other agencies' efforts to identify technologies) sources will provide later warning, perhaps in some cases only after the introduction of the technology, but greater detail and more accurate predictions of its likely impact. There is some overlap between these categories. For example, experts at the cutting edge may also act as *primary* information sources.

Thus the choice of information sources requires a trade-off between earlier warning and greater accuracy. Early sources, which include patents, notification of phase I trials, conference abstracts, and pharmaceutical and biotechnology companies give early warning but with poor specificity (in that they can yield a large number of false positives) and uncertainty about the technology's likely impact, its precise application, or the timing of its introduction. Later sources, which include leading articles in key medical journals, licensing applications, and newsletters and bulletins from other agencies provide very clear and precise information of a given technology with high sensitivity and specificity but relatively late warning to the health system.

The relative importance of each of the sources depends upon the type of innovation under consideration. Clearly, some technologies are easier to identify than others. Formal registration, regulatory monitoring systems, and the publication of the results of phase I–III studies make drugs the easiest. For example, dornase alfa for cystic fibrosis could have been tracked through a series of publications from 1992.[23–26] Nevertheless little has been done until recently to use such intelligence as part of an early warning system.

The case studies suggest that particularly important documentary sources include key pharmaceutical journals, specialist medical journals (defined as those journals which contain case reports and case series which strongly influence early adopters) and Food and Drug Administration licensing applications in the USA. For example, there were numerous early reports on beta interferon in journals in the early and mid 1980s.[27–30] Conference reports can also be useful – laparoscopic cholecystectomy underwent rapid diffusion after innovators presented videotapes at surgical society meetings in the United States in 1989.[31] The introduction of donepezil in the UK during the 1990s illustrates the opportunities that existed to identify this drug before it was licensed and the potential benefits that may have resulted from such early warning (Box 19.4).

Although the Delphi survey identified experts as only one of a number of important sources, existing systems reported that liaison with experts is essential. It allows access to informal networks in a particular field that can communicate research findings by personal contact before they have been published.[17] Informal networks also identify gaps, give a flavour of the importance of technologies and provide insight into changing technologies. Telemedicine would

221

Box 19.4 Donepezil for dementia of the Alzheimer's type in the UK

Donepezil (Aricept) is a drug for mild to moderate dementia due to senile dementia of the Alzheimer's type which was licensed world-wide during 1996 and 1997. Before donepezil, very little was available for the treatment of dementia. Marketing of donepezil has focused on specialist services, although it can be prescribed in primary care.

At the higher dose preparation the cost per patient per year of donepezil is approximately £1200 (1997). There are approximately 240 000 potential recipients living in the United Kingdom; a potential cost of £288 million per year. Potential savings are uncertain.

There were numerous opportunities to identify donepezil: animal studies can be traced back to 1980 and the early 1990s saw the publication of a number of studies in specialist medical journals. However, at the time of the drug's introduction there had been only three randomised trials, of which only one had been published in full. The debate about the cost-effectiveness of donepezil continued after licensing.[32]

One of the difficulties in establishing the effectiveness of donepezil in routine clinical practice has been the lack of accurate measures of the quality of life of dementia patients. Early warning in the early–mid 1980s of the host of drugs in development for dementia could have provided the impetus for the development of such measures. This may have enabled a more rational introduction of these drugs into clinical practice, possibly as part of randomised trials incorporating the refined measure. Early warning could also have enabled more timely preparation of prescribing guidelines.

---

have been relatively easy to identify as a potentially important new health care technology at virtually any time over the past 30 years given the large capital outlay and organisational implications of this technology and its marketing by manufacturers. However, watchful waiting for technological developments in other fields and the appropriate organisational environment, with the aid of experts, was required in order to predict when telemedicine's diffusion would become widespread. Similarly, biosensor research began in the 1950s and 1960s but the history of the development of such devices has been closely related to advances in biotechnology, materials science, and electronics. Thus, the development and likely use of biosensors *per se* would have been relatively easy to predict a long time ago but commercial secrecy and uncertainty[33] would have meant that it would not have been straightforward to predict when, and precisely which, biosensors would begin to make a real impact on health services.

Recommendations

The establishment of an early warning system is a new concept for virtually all countries. Such a system is usually part of a health technology assessment programme and seeks to help control and rationalise the complex patterns of adoption and diffusion of technologies that are being promoted by the health care industry and professional opinion leaders. It may also take a longer term perspective and be used alongside industry to develop desirable technologies.

An ideal early warning system would take heed of the suggestions from the case studies, Delphi survey and existing systems. Iteration between the use of documentary sources and the involvement of experts is vital, and consequently a combination of the following information sources (many of which can now be accessed via the Internet) is recommended:

- scanning of key pharmaceutical journals, specialist medical journals, key medical journals, Food and Drug Administration licensing applications, and conference abstracts to produce a database of potential technologies;
- liaison with pharmaceutical and biotechnology companies, and medical engineering companies; and
- regular meetings and/or surveys involving sentinel groups of expert health professionals.

Such a system, established at a national level, could help in the preparation of guidelines for purchasers and providers of health care in advance of the introduction of new innovations, estimations of future expenditure implications, and establishment of national priorities for research on cost-effectiveness, thereby enabling an iterative approach to the evaluation of innovations to be put in place. These applications of early warning will help to minimise unnecessary costs, health disbenefits, and policy confusion.

References

1. Drummond MF. Economic evaluation and the rational diffusion and use of health technology. *Health Policy* 1987;7:309–24.

2. Department of Health. *Report of the NHS Health Technology Assessment Programme 1995*. London: HMSO, 1995.
3. Peckham M. Towards research based health care. In: Newsom-Davis J, Weatherall D (eds), *Health policy and technological innovation*. London: The Royal Society, 1994.
4. Smith L, McClenahan J. *Management of the introduction of Betaferon. A Developmental Evaluation*. London: Kings Fund, 1997.
5. Cuschieri A. Whither minimal access surgery: tribulations and expectations. *Am J Surg* 1995;**169**:9–19.
6. Bonair A, Perrson J. Innovation and diffusion of health care technologies. In: Szczepura A, Kankaanpaa J (eds), *Assessment of health care technologies. Case studies, key concepts and strategic issues*, Cambridge: John Wiley & Sons, 1996.
7. Rogers EM. *Diffusion of innovations*. New York: Free Press, Macmillan, 4th edn, 1995.
8. Luiten AL. The birth and development of an innovation: the case of magnetic resonance imaging. In: Rutten FFH, Reiser SJ (eds), *The economics of medical technology. Proceedings of an international conference on economics of medical technology*, Berlin: Springer-Verlag, 1988.
9. Battelle. *Analysis of selected biomedical research programs. Volume 2*. Columbus, Ohio: Battelle Columbus Laboratories, 1976.
10. Gelijns AC. *Innovations in clinical practice, the dynamics of medical technology development*. Washington DC: National Academy Press, 1991.
11. Banta HD, Gelijns AC. The future and healthcare technology: implications of a system for early identification. *World Health Statist Quart* 1994;**47**:140–8.
12. Sculpher M, Drummond M, Buxton M. The iterative use of economic evaluation as part of the process of health technology assessment. *J Health Serv Res Policy* 1997;**2**:26–30.
13. Smee C. The need for early warning in health policy making and planning. In: *European workshop: Scanning the horizon for emerging health technologies*, Copenhagen, 1997.
14. Food & Drug Administration. *Forecast of emerging technologies*. Rockville, MD: Food & Drug Administration, 1981.
15. Spiby J. Advances in medical technology over the next twenty years. *Community Med* 1988;**10**:273–8.
16. Banta HD, Gelijns AC, Griffioen J, Graaff PJ. An inquiry concerning future healthcare technology: methods and general results. *Health Policy* 1987;**8**: 251–64.
17. Steering Committee on Future Health Scenarios. *Anticipating and assessing health care technology. Volume 1: general considerations and policy conclusions*. Zoetermeer, The Netherlands: Martinus Nijhoff, 1987.
18. Mowatt G, Bower DJ, Brebner JA, Cairns JA, Grant AM, McKee L. When and how to assess fast-changing technologies: a comparative study of medical applications of four generic technologies. *Health Technol Assess* 1997;**1** (14).
19. Stevens A, Packer C, Robert G. Early warning of new health care technologies in the United Kingdom. *Int J Technol Assess Health Care* (in press).
20. Stevens A, Robert G, Gabbay J. Identifying new health care technologies in the United Kingdom. *Int J Technol Assess Health Care* 1997;**13**:59–67.
21. Technology Foresight. *Progress through partnership 4. Health & life sciences panel*. London: Office of Science and Technology, 1995.
22. Department of Health. *Report of Genetics Research Advisory Group*. London: HMSO, 1995.
23. Hubbard RC, McElvaney NG, Birrer P *et al*. A preliminary study of aerosolized recombinant human deoxyribonuclease I in the treatment of cystic fibrosis. *New Engl J Med* 1992;**326**:812–15.

24. Aitken ML, Burke W, McDonald G, Shak S, Bruce Montgomery A, Smith A. Recombinant human DNAse inhalation in normal subjects and patients with cystic fibrosis. *J Am Med Assoc* 1992;**267**:1947–51.
25. Ranasinha C, Assoufi B, Shak S *et al.* Efficacy and safety of short-term administration of aerosolized recombinant human DNAse I in adults with stable stage cystic fibrosis. *Lancet* 1993;**324**:199–202.
26. Fuchs HJ, Borowitz DS, Christiansen DH *et al.* Effect of aerosolized recombinant human DNAse on exacerbations of respiratory symptoms and on pulmonary function in patients with cystic fibrosis. *New Engl J Med* 1994;**331**: 637–42.
27. Jacobs L, O'Malley J, Freeman A *et al.* Intrathecal interferon in multiple sclerosis. *Arch Neurol* 1982;**39**:609–15.
28. Jacobs L, O'Malley J, Freeman A *et al.* Intrathecal interferon in multiple sclerosis. Patient follow-up. *Arch Neurol* 1985;**42**:841–7.
29. Jacobs L, Salazar AM, Herndon R *et al.* Intrathecally administered natural human fibroblast interferon reduces exacerbations of multiple sclerosis. Results of a multicenter, double-blind study. *Arch Neurol* 1987;**44**:589–95.
30. McFarlin DE. Use of interferon in multiple sclerosis. *Ann Neurol* 1985;**18**: 432–3.
31. Gelijns AC, Rosenberg N. The dynamics of innovation in minimally invasive therapy. *Health Policy* 1993;**23**:153–66.
32. Donepezil for Alzheimer's Disease? *Drugs Therap Bull* 1997;**35**:75–6.
33. Schultz JS. Biosensors. *Sci Am* 1991;(Aug):48–55.

20 Evaluating new and fast-changing technologies

D JANE BOWER, GRAHAM MOWATT,
JOHN A BREBNER, JOHN A CAIRNS,
ADRIAN M GRANT AND LORNA McKEE

This chapter provides insights into factors influencing timing and choice of methods of assessment of new and fast-changing technologies.[1] While observations are made about health technology assessment (HTA) in general, our recommendations are based on the situation in the United Kingdom.

Health technologies have been broadly defined as including any method used by health professionals to promote health, prevent and treat disease, and improve rehabilitation and long-term care.[2] HTA is the evaluation of the benefits and costs (clinical, social, economic, and system-wide) of transferring a technology into clinical practice.[3] There is currently no accepted formula for the timing of the assessment of new and fast-evolving technologies. By their nature, they are often difficult to evaluate by accepted methods.

An additional problem is posed by the growing diversity of decision-makers involved in new technology adoption. Depending on a number of factors, such as the amount of controversy surrounding a generic technology (for example, genetic manipulation), decision-making may be subject on the one hand to central monitoring or statutory regulation or, on the other hand, to some degree of decentralisation and absence of regulation. Apart from ethical pharmaceuticals, routine systems have not yet been devised for evaluation and control of many other types of interventions that have obvious potential for harm.[4]

Nature of the evidence

A series of literature searches was undertaken in an attempt to identify papers focusing on, firstly, the general principles involved in timing of health technology assessments, and secondly, reported assessments of six specific medical applications:

- laparoscopic cholecystectomy
- chorion villus sampling
- teleradiology
- teledermatology
- genetic screening for predisposition to breast cancer, and
- gene therapy for cystic fibrosis.

The reported assessments were analysed in order to try to identify factors which influenced the timing of these assessments. The six medical applications offered a number of useful paired comparisons, for example between those which were "tele-" or "chromosome-" based, and between those which were new/evolving and those relatively well-established (Table 20.1). Since the

Table 20.1   The six medical applications reviewed and their generic technologies

Generic technology	Application
Karyotyping	Chorion villus sampling
Minimal access surgery	Cholecystectomy
Genetic manipulation	Gene therapy (cystic fibrosis)
	Diagnosis of genetic susceptibility to breast cancer
Videoconferencing (telemedicine)	Radiology
	Dermatology

literature relating to the six applications gave only a limited indication as to the timing of the assessments, a number of interviews with key individuals were undertaken. This provided important additional insights.

A bibliometric study of publication trends in the six applications was also undertaken in an attempt to identify points in the development of a technology which could be used as crude indicators that assessment should be initiated. Figure 20.1 shows, for the period 1970–1995, the number of references each year identified from a MEDLINE search for each of the six medical

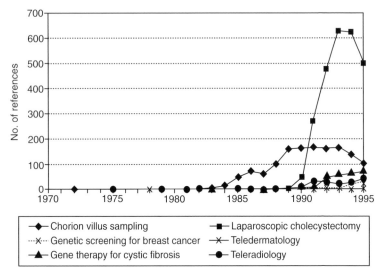

Figure 20.1   Number of references in MEDLINE for six technologies (1970–1995).

applications. While annual numbers of references for the relatively established applications of laparoscopic cholecystectomy and chorion villus sampling appear to have peaked and are now declining, those for the remaining four applications, although far fewer in number, are continuing to increase.

Findings

The consensus that emerged from the review on timing was that assessments should be initiated early,[5-7] that they should employ a variety of approaches in order to overcome some of the problems associated with each method,[8] and that they should be iterative.[9] Randomisation of the first sick patient to receive a new drug or undergo a new procedure was advocated by some writers.[10] However, the existence of finite resources for health technology assessment means that it is not feasible to evaluate all new health technologies through randomised controlled trials (RCTs). Indeed, randomised trials might sometimes be unnecessary, inadequate, or even impossible.[11] For instance, where a technology has a large, demonstrable impact, non-randomised studies might be sufficient.

An important point that arose in relation to economic impact evaluations was the difficulty of reliably predicting the pattern of demand when a new technology became available. This was particularly evident in the case of minimal access surgery, where substantial capital and training investment was already being made on the basis of earlier predictions that most surgery was expected to use this approach within the next few years.[12,13] More recent evaluations of laparoscopic cholecystectomy gave less positive results than earlier studies.[14] Telemedicine applications were also expected to change the pattern of demand, but the economic impact would depend on how service delivery was modified to deal with it.

Are the methods in use adequate for new, fast-changing technologies?

There were questions as to whether the methods in use were adequate for every technology. HTA traditionally focused on clinical outcomes. Now there are demands for a much wider range of criteria to be addressed including social and ethical impact, and the effect on patterns of demand for health care.

Best practice employed a number of methods, rigorously applied and reported, in order to achieve the most satisfactory outcomes for patients, but even in combination none of these methods was foolproof. Rare side effects were often only detected after extensive use. New problems could arise due to the different ethical and cultural concerns of different patient groups.

The problems with assessing the four fast-changing technologies were not qualitatively different; they were just likely to arise more frequently during the development phase of a technology. Cystic fibrosis gene therapy was being developed under tight central regulation comparable to drugs.[15,16] If approved, it would be used in an extremely constrained fashion. Any changes would have to be subjected to extensive testing. In contrast, genetic diagnostic testing for breast cancer susceptibility, a non-invasive procedure, was being regulated less tightly, but with tight control on diffusion.[17,18] Also, telemedicine was only beginning to be assessed on a limited basis, and there were no controls on adoption. This was a function of its low risk profile in the eyes of users. Thus the approaches to assessment were more a function of perceived risk than of rate of change. The

229

methods in use were not in themselves more inadequate than for more stable technologies.

How and when have assessments been carried out?

The timing of assessments often reflected the growth of either clinical concern about side effects (laparoscopic cholecystectomy, chorion villus sampling), political concern about being seen to do something (cystic fibrosis gene therapy, genetic diagnosis) or growing popular demand/concern (genetic technologies). In some of these cases, such as laparoscopic cholecystectomy, this meant that assessment was not initiated until it proved "too late" to carry out a large-scale RCT comparing laparoscopic with open cholecystectomy.[19] Laparoscopic cholecystectomy also illustrated the difficulty of achieving properly randomised trials when public interest has been aroused and a popular consensus about a procedure has been formed.[20] Thus media coverage of a health technology, and/or physician influence, might engender patient reluctance to participate in a randomised trial.

In the case of cystic fibrosis gene therapy and chorion villus sampling, an early decision to assess allowed effective control and thorough assessment approaches to be used.[21-26] However, the highly regulated cystic fibrosis randomised trials now underway are costly and slow. This highly precautionary approach is acceptable for invasive or otherwise risky applications but it might be difficult to justify imposing such regulation on innovations that were not perceived by clinicians or the public to have adverse potential. Where an application is neither invasive nor seen to have alarming implications for health-related aspects of the patient's life, it would be hard to impose expensive regulatory control. Telemedicine applications, for instance, would currently be unlikely to arouse sufficient concern. However, this *laissez-faire* approach might prove to be misguided if there was, for example, misdiagnosis using telemedicine leading to harm and successful litigation. In contrast to telemedicine, genetic testing, with its implications for life insurance and other important matters, was widely perceived as requiring some regulation and control. Thus public and clinical perception of the risks associated with an application was very important in determining whether assessment was undertaken early enough to be effective. This argued for greater education and debate about these issues.

230

Are there lessons to be learnt from the applications which have now reached a relatively stable state, that could be applied to the fast-evolving technologies?

Where assessment was initiated early and systematically, as with chorion villus sampling, the initial study and subsequent work have provided a more useful and comprehensible body of information to guide decisions. Where assessment was initiated late, after some diffusion had taken place, as with laparoscopic cholecystectomy, the studies were less satisfactory and rigorous, and interpretation of data was not easy.

Another point which became evident with both of the "stable" technologies was that although the rate of publication of evaluations had fallen off, studies were still being published which either conflicted with earlier studies (laparoscopic cholecystectomy)[27,28] or added important data (chorion villus sampling).[29,30] They were not, in fact, entirely stable, although the rate of development had fallen to a low level. It is probable that health technologies continue to evolve until they are clearly superseded.

Is it possible to draw any inferences about trends in development/diffusion of technologies from collective characteristics of reported assessments, which can be used to decide on timing of assessments?

The bibliometric study covered too few applications to give a clear indication as to whether this might be an approach which would yield useful indicator points to trigger HTAs. In addition some applications had such a limited literature that the absolute numbers of publications were too small to use in this way. However the laparoscopic cholecystectomy (Figure 20.2) and chorion villus sampling (Figure 20.3) publication trend curves gave more promising inflection points, at times approximating to dates at which assessment should have been initiated. This was suggestive, although the results were too limited to generalise from.

Figure 20.2 shows, for the period 1989–1995, the number of references each year identified from a MEDLINE search for laparoscopic cholecystectomy. The number of references per year, represented by columns, is set against the main RCTs of laparoscopic versus open cholecystectomy, and laparoscopic versus minicholecystectomy, represented by horizontal lines. One

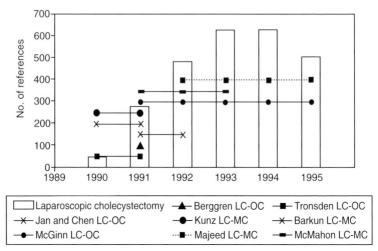

Figure 20.2 Number of references each year, identified from MEDLINE, for laparoscopic cholecystectomy (1989–1995) and the duration of the major clinical trials.

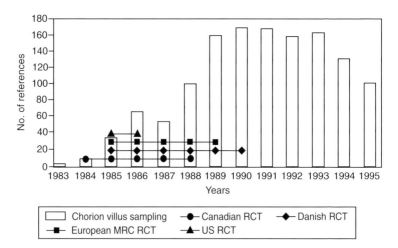

Figure 20.3 Number of references each year, identified from MEDLINE, for chorion villus sampling (1983–1995) and the duration of the major clinical trials.

reference appeared in 1989, followed by a dramatic increase in numbers over the next few years, peaking at over 600 references per year for 1993 and 1994, with 1995 appearing to signal a decline in numbers. It can be seen, therefore, that over a relatively short period of time, a significant amount of publishing activity was generated on the subject of laparoscopic cholecystectomy.

Figure 20.3 shows, for the period 1983–1995, the number of references each year identified from a MEDLINE search for chorion villus sampling. The number of references per year, represented by columns, is set against the main studies which took place of chorion villus sampling versus amniocentesis, represented by horizontal lines. The first references appeared in 1983, with annual numbers on the whole steadily increasing until peaking over the period 1989–1993, followed by a decline in 1994–1995.

Figures 20.2 and 20.3 suggest that there may be a brief "window of opportunity" when it is possible to initiate a randomised trial of a new procedure. This "window" may open from around the time that the first papers on a new procedure appear in the clinical literature. It may close when coverage in the clinical literature and the wider media has sufficiently influenced both clinicians' and patients' views to reduce any perceived uncertainty about the procedure's safety and effectiveness.

Guidelines for assessment

It would be helpful to categorise technologies into, for instance, diagnostic versus therapeutic, and invasive versus non-invasive. It would be more feasible to provide a set of protocols for each category than to try to derive a very general code applicable to all. The form of such protocols could be a flow diagram, containing a series of questions and directions, to assist decision-makers in determining whether they should undertake assessment or refer to appropriate national bodies for guidance, what form assessment should take, and reporting rules. Such protocols could only be created after agreement on standard assessment and reporting procedures was reached. A strongly precautionary approach would clearly be appropriate for the more invasive, ethically problematic and costly technologies. A technology might be assigned a score on each of several parameters and the overall total used to decide on priorities for evaluation. A series of different tests could be applied depending on the initial score, to decide on the next step. Provided the guidelines were sufficiently clear, this would allow local commissioners of health services and ethics committees to decide whether they were competent

233

to evaluate a new technology, or whether they should refer to central authority for further guidance.

Standardisation would be doubly useful because it would facilitate meta-analysis of studies. It emerged from the literature reviewed that there had been little attempt in many cases to make studies comparable to what had been done before.

Recommendations

A further series of bibliometric studies of a wider range of literature would be valuable in order to explore the possibility of using inflections in trend curves as indicators of when to initiate assessment. Women's media could be included in the range of literature reviewed since, in the case of chorion villus sampling and breast cancer diagnosis, the role of consumer pressure was evident.

The literature illustrates the very diverse characteristics of different health care technologies and the problems associated with a single methodological approach. Given their diversity, it is unlikely that a global theory of HTA will be suited to all, although there are clearly some important common principles. However, these relate more to the demands for relative safety and effectiveness, rather than to a stereotypical protocol for the timing or nature of assessment.

A first step towards addressing this issue would be to reduce the complexity of any one case somewhat by categorising health technologies on the basis of, for example, their invasiveness and of possible characteristics such as their apparent cost advantages or disadvantages, their potential for major improvements to public health, and their ethical impact. The question of which methods of evaluation to apply and when to apply them would be easier to answer when the category of health technology was more precisely defined and its risk characteristics assessed.

References

1. Mowatt G, Bower DJ, Brebner JA, Cairns JA, Grant AM, McKee L. When and how to assess fast-changing technologies: a comparative study of medical applications of four generic technologies. *Health Technol Assess* 1997;1(14): 1–149.
2. Standing Group on Health Technology. *1994 Annual Report*. London: Department of Health, 1995.

3. Russell I. *Can it work? Does it work? Research design for health technology assessment.* York: University of York, 1996.
4. Gelijns AC. *Modern methods of clinical investigation.* Washington: National Academy Press, 1990.
5. Department of Health. *Assessing the effects of health technologies: principles, practice, proposals.* London: Department of Health, 1992.
6. Gelijns A, Rosenberg N. The dynamics of technological change in medicine. *Health Aff* 1994;**13**(3):28–46.
7. Banta HD. Dutch committee assesses the future of health technology. *Dimensions Health Service* 1986;**63**(7):17–20.
8. Franklin C. Basic concepts and fundamental issues in technology assessment. *Intensive Care Med* 1993;**19**:117–21.
9. Banta HD, Andreasen PB. The political dimension in health care technology assessment programs. *Int J Technol Assess Health Care* 1990;**6**:115–23.
10. Chalmers TC. Randomisation of the first patient. *Med Clin North Am* 1975; **59**:1035–8.
11. Black N. Why we need observational studies to evaluate the effectiveness of health care. *Br Med J* 1996;**312**:1215–18.
12. Cuschieri A. *Minimal access surgery: implications for the NHS. Report from a Working Group chaired by Professor Alfred Cuschieri.* Edinburgh: HMSO, 1994.
13. Border P. *Minimal access ("keyhole") surgery and its implications.* London: Parliamentary Office of Science and Technology, 1995.
14. Downs SH, Black NA, Devlin HB, Royston CMS, Russell RCG. Systematic review of the effectiveness and safety of laparoscopic cholecystectomy. *Ann Roy Coll Surg Engl* 1996;**78**:235–323.
15. Caplen NJ, Gao X, Hayes P *et al.* Gene therapy for cystic fibrosis in humans by liposome-mediated DNA transfer: the production of resources and the regulatory process. *Gene Therapy* 1994;**1**:139–47.
16. Zallen DT. Public oversight is necessary if human gene therapy is to progress. *Hum Gene Ther* 1996;**7**:795–7.
17. Josefson D. US doctors warned about test for breast cancer gene. *Br Med J* 1996;**312**:1057–8.
18. Stix G. Is genetic testing premature? *Sci Am* 1996;**275**(3):73.
19. Macintyre IMC, Wilson RG. Laparoscopic cholecystectomy. *Br J Surg* 1993; **80**:552–9.
20. Sculpher M. *A snip at the price? A review of the economics of minimal access surgery.* Uxbridge: Brunel University, 1993.
21. Zabner J, Couture LA, Gregory RJ, Graham SM, Smith AE, Welsh MJ. Adenovirus-mediated gene transfer transiently corrects the chloride transport defect in nasal epithelia of patients with cystic fibrosis. *Cell* 1993;**75**:207–16.
22. Crystal RG, McElvaney NG, Rosenfeld MA *et al.* Administration of an adenovirus containing the human CFTR cDNA to the respiratory tract of individuals with cystic fibrosis. *Nat Genet* 1994;**8**:42–51.
23. Knowles MR, Hohneker KW, Zhou Z *et al.* A controlled study of adenoviral-vector-mediated gene transfer in the nasal epithelium of patients with cystic fibrosis. *New Engl J Med* 1995;**333**:823–31.
24. Lippman A, Tomkins DJ, Shime J, Hamerton JL. Canadian multicentre randomized clinical trial of chorion villus sampling and amniocentesis. Final report. *Prenat Diagn* 1992;**12**:385–408.
25. MRC Working Party on the evaluation of chorion villus sampling. Medical Research Council European Trial of chorion villus sampling. *Lancet* 1991;**337**: 1491–9.
26. Smidt-Jensen S, Permin M, Philip J *et al.* Randomised comparison of amniocentesis and transabdominal and transcervical chorionic villus sampling. *Lancet* 1992;**340**:1237–44.

27. McGinn FP, Miles AJG, Uglow M, Ozmen M, Terzi C, Humby M. Randomised trial of laparoscopic cholecystectomy and minicholecystectomy. *Br J Surg* 1995; **82**:1374–7.
28. Majeed AW, Troy G, Nicholl JP *et al*. Randomised, prospective, single-blind comparison of laparoscopic versus small-incision cholecystectomy. *Lancet* 1996; **347**:989–94.
29. Firth HV, Boyd PA, Chamberlain P, MacKenzie IZ, Lindenbaum RH, Huson SM. Severe limb abnormalities after chorion villus sampling at 56–66 days' gestation. *Lancet* 1991;**337**:762–3.
30. Burton BK, Schulz CJ, Burd LI. Limb anomalies associated with chorionic villus sampling. *Obstet Gynecol* 1992;**79**:726–30.

21 Research implementation methods

NICK FREEMANTLE, MARTIN ECCLES,
JAMES MASON, MARY ANN THOMSON,
FREDERICK M WOLF AND JOHN WOOD

Research produces many findings which, if implemented, will benefit patients. However, the availability of such findings has led to the realisation that research does not, automatically, diffuse into practice.[1] Increasingly the findings of research are summarised in clinical practice guidelines and a new industry has appeared, concerned with their development and implementation.

Alongside these developments, there has been considerable interest in developing suitable approaches for implementation, such as computerised prompts or modern approaches to education, as well as interest in evaluating their effectiveness and cost-effectiveness. Although a great deal is known about the design of randomised[2] and non-randomised studies,[3] there remains a considerable amount to learn about the application of these approaches in the field of implementation research.

Nature of the evidence

This chapter describes the main findings of a review of implementation methods. It was not our intention to produce a consensus document reflecting the breadth of beliefs among people working in this area, but to derive recommendations based upon empirical evidence where it was available, or derived from first principles.

We attempted to locate empirically based methodological articles while developing a database of evaluations of implementation studies[4] using searches of MEDLINE and Embase, a hand search of the journal *Medical Care* (which contains a high yield of relevant research) and from existing bibliographies. With the exception of two studies examining the appropriateness of analyses conducted in implementation trials,[5,6] no empirically based methodological studies were located, although we did accumulate a number of articles which described authors' opinions on how such research should be conducted. These highlighted a number of important methodological issues:

- when to use comparative studies to evaluate implementation methods;
- the appropriateness of different study designs;
- the design of economic evaluations in implementation studies;
- the appropriate unit of analysis in implementation studies; and
- the state of the art in summarising the findings of a series of implementation studies.

Findings

When to use comparative study designs

Formal evaluation in some form of comparative study is essential to evaluate appropriately an implementation method. For example, in an evaluation of the impact of evidence-based guidelines on the appropriateness of caesarean section, Lomas *et al.*[7] describe how a third of obstetricians reported changing their practice in the light of the guideline, when the guideline actually led to only a 0·13% attributable reduction in the overall rate of caesarean section.

We also found examples where researchers had perhaps moved too hastily to undertake comparative studies. For example, the perceived need for information by primary care physicians was identified in one small trial measuring clinician knowledge,[8] and then its provision subsequently evaluated within a larger randomised trial with objective measures of patient and health professional outcomes, rather than knowledge alone.[9] The trial showed that the simple provision of information to doctors did not, unfortunately, appear to bring substantial direct benefits to patients, a conclusion confirmed in a subsequent systematic review of this question.[10] In a participant observational study, Covell *et al.*[11] found that the perceived need for better information among office-based practitioners was not reflected in their behaviour. Although doctors perceived that they answered questions that arose in their work from traditional information sources such as textbooks and journal articles, they actually resolved such issues through consultation with colleagues. It was, *a priori*, highly unlikely that the provision of information by itself would be effective. In other words, the quantitative evaluation was ill-focused when considered in the light of the relevant qualitative research. Thus, although ultimately evaluation using comparative studies is important when evaluating promising implementation methods, this should not be conducted before appropriate development work has been undertaken, to assess the feasibility of an intervention, and a plausible taxonomy for the mechanism through which the intended behavioural change will be achieved has been developed.[12] There has been considerable theoretical and practical study of the diffusion of innovation and change outside the realms of medicine,[13] but it is not clear that those involved in health services research have as yet appropriately considered these issues.

The appropriateness of different comparative study designs

It has been argued that simple randomised trials may not be the most appropriate designs for evaluating implementation interventions. Instead, complex designs such as Latin Squares[14] have been advocated, although these have been used only rarely. The replicated Latin Square design, used in the North of England Study of Standards in General Practice,[15] combines not only different clinical topics (for example itchy rash or bedwetting) with different groups of GPs, but also different interventions (for example audit and feedback or local standard setting), in order to examine the interaction of different factors. Also, it has been advocated that non-randomised studies may provide useful information (see Chapters 6 and 7). These are studies in which allocation to comparator groups is other than by chance (random) or, in the case of interrupted time series, the comparison is with historical trends.

The well known advantage of allocation by a chance process is that differences between groups in a randomised evaluation reflect only the effects, if any, of an intervention and the play of chance. This simplifies analysis and attribution considerably. The problems with non-random allocation may be illustrated by an interesting Swiss study of mass media interventions which focused on the use of hysterectomy.[16] Although the annual rate of hysterectomy decreased after the mass media campaign in the Canton of Ticino, the year before the intervention had also been accompanied by a small decrease (Figure 21.1). The neighbouring Canton of Bern

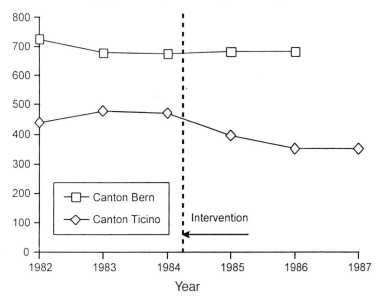

Figure 21.1   Hysterectomy rates per 100 000 women in two Swiss cantons (1982–1987).[16]

had experienced a fall in its rate between 1982 and 1983 for which no explanation is offered. Also, rather than being responsible for change, the mass media campaign, which was sparked by an article by the chief surgeon of a public hospital, may have reflected concern among clinicians that was already leading to a change in the intervention rate. Without random allocation it is not possible to attribute cause and effect with certainty. The investigators statement that "there seems to be no doubt that the decrease in hysterectomies in Ticino was the result of the mass media information campaign", seems overstated.

The problems with non-randomised studies makes randomisation appropriate when it is feasible, and there are at least 200 randomised trials that examine implementation methods.[4] More complex designs, particularly Latin Squares, do not appear to have substantial advantages, as it is rare that an appropriate mix of subjects, interventions, and topics will be available and, perhaps more fundamentally, the existing examples in the literature do not provide results that are readily interpretable. Row and column designs, in which subjects are randomised to one of a range of discrete interventions, do appear helpful in many situations where examining different attributes of an intervention may be considered desirable (for example, examining the effects of disseminating guidelines covering different clinical areas). Importantly, however, there will be situations where random allocation is simply not feasible (for example in mass media campaigns, or national guidelines implementation programmes) but evaluation is still clearly desirable, in which case use of non-randomised designs (particularly interrupted time series) may provide useful information.

Appropriate outcomes

The outcome of interest in implementation studies is normally a change in the behaviour of a health professional, rather than a change in patients' health status. Conducting implementation trials is probably unethical before a valid and worthwhile message has been identified. This being the case, the implementation trial evaluates the extent to which behaviour can be changed to achieve the benefits of the message. Treatment guidelines for implementation are often derived from large-scale randomised trials and, if over 2000 patients are required to provide evidence of effectiveness for angiotensin converting enzyme inhibitors, it seems most unlikely that a trial of an educational intervention that aims to implement such findings will be able to estimate such treatment effects with adequate precision.

Patient outcome measures may be argued for in implementation trials where there is concern that benefits from randomised trials may not translate into local practice, or to ensure that an untoward effect of treatment is not occurring. However, a pragmatic treatment trial is likely to be more appropriate (that is the worthwhile nature of intervention has yet to be fully established), and data on patient outcomes collected in such studies are unlikely to provide valid insights into the effects of an intervention.

Economic evaluations in implementation studies

Considering the costs of achieving change alongside the benefits is just as important in implementation studies as in clinical studies (see Chapter 3). Appropriately conducted economic analyses may provide relevant policy recommendations to decision-makers. In spite of the importance of economic analyses in this area, we are not aware of an adequate example of such an economic analysis in the published literature.

The appropriate unit of analysis in implementation studies

The unit of analysis refers to the level at which differences in effects are modelled in a study. Decisions on the unit of analysis are closely related to decisions on the unit of randomisation. In clinical studies, the appropriate unit of analysis is often quite straightforward, as patients are the target of the intervention and improvement in their health status is the desired outcome. Thus, patients provide the natural unit of analysis. Where patient outcome may be affected by extraneous factors, such as treatment in a particular centre, it is common for this to be taken into account at the design and analysis stage.

In implementation studies, the appropriateness of the unit of analysis has been frequently ignored.[5,6] At its worst, this has meant that although practitioners have been targeted, patients have provided the unit of analysis. Where there are a large number of patients treated by a relatively small number of practitioners, this can lead to a misleading increase in statistical power and in some circumstances also affect the estimate of effect.[17]

Some investigators have advocated the use of cluster randomisation in order to increase the apparent statistical power in implementation trials (see Chapter 11). This can involve taking patients as the unit of analysis but taking account of the observed intracluster correlation coefficient,[18–21] a measure of the degree to which patients are related to their treatment setting. However, this approach will only be appropriate if a statistical analysis conducted at the patient level makes sense initially. Where a study is intervening with health professionals, and it is their behaviour that is targeted, analysis of patients as if they were primarily the group of interest will provide misleadingly tight confidence intervals that may only be partly corrected through using the cluster randomisation approach.

Where it is appropriate to analyse in this way, the estimated intrapractice correlation coefficient is also open to measurement error and it is important that this is taken into account, perhaps through sensitivity analysis using the 95% confidence intervals of the correlation coefficient.

Selecting an appropriate unit of analysis in an implementation study is not straightforward, and experts get it wrong surprisingly regularly. Some questions that may guide an appropriate choice are contained in Box 21.1. As a rule of thumb, if you are concerned

---

Box 21.1 Questions to inform decisions on an appropriate unit of analysis

1. What is the unit of randomisation?
2. At what level is the intervention aimed (e.g. doctors, patients, hospitals)?
3. What is the main outcome being measured?
4. What are the major factors that affect results (other than the interventions themselves)?

---

that there may be important differences between subjects who are at a higher level than the unit of analysis (for example in a trial that is providing education for doctors who work closely together in practices with shared formularies), it is important that the analysis takes this into account, and that there are sufficient practices in the study to enable a robust estimate of the variation between them.

Overviews of implementation studies

The last few years have seen a considerable advance in methods to synthesise the results from randomised trials (see Chapter 16). This has led not only to a greater understanding of the methods but also concern about their overinterpretation.[22-24] Quantitative synthesis has historically been used to combine the results of randomised trials in related areas, such as education.[25] We reviewed available methods and concluded that a good quality, systematic review of implementation studies should attempt to assess thoroughly the quality and context of relevant studies (so called "narrative review") and use appropriate statistical methods to provide estimates of the likelihood that the results observed may have occurred by chance, with confidence intervals to describe the likely range of values. Such approaches may enable the quantitative examination of factors that may explain differences between study results[23] using regression models, and quantitative estimation of the degree to which a review may be open to publication bias using the "file drawer" method.[25] A thoughtful and non-mechanistic use of both approaches, narrative and quantitative, will aid a valid and reliable interpretation of available studies.

We made a systematic review of the methods used in reviews of implementation studies located through a search of MEDLINE. None of the 18 reviews that we identified (including some to which we had contributed) used an optimal combination of quantitative and narrative review techniques. The crude and potentially biased technique of vote counting of statistically significant studies[26] is, however, commonly employed. Reviewers rarely state how they dealt with the appropriateness of units of analysis in studies included or the interpretation of multiple outcome measures relating to a common underlying effect in studies. They do, however, frequently make strong concluding statements on the effectiveness of interventions on the basis of narrative reviews and vote counting methods. In fact, it was often rather difficult to see how conclusions were derived. Interestingly, the reviews which had used appropriate quantitative methods tended to furnish more cautious conclusions.

Recommendations

Implementing research findings is an important issue, but the science of evaluating different implementation methods is still at an early stage. Our review led to the following recommendations.

- Although evaluation using comparative studies is important, this should not be conducted before appropriate development work has been undertaken to assess the feasibility of an intervention, and to develop a plausible social model.
- Where practical, random allocation to different groups should be used. Where this is not possible, non-randomised methods, particularly interrupted time series, enable some formal evaluation of the effects of an intervention.
- Implementation will normally focus upon changes in professional practice rather than patient outcome.

- Economic evaluation should be conducted in implementation studies.
- An appropriate unit of analysis should be used.
- Reviews of implementation studies should use an appropriate mix of quantitative and narrative methods upon which to base their conclusions.

There are also more general conclusions that apply across areas but are nonetheless important. In particular, the problems of publication bias and poor reporting are not limited to clinical studies[27] and may be particularly important when interventions themselves are inadequately described.

References

1. Antman EM, Lau J, Kupelnick B, Mosteller F, Chalmers TC. A comparison of results of meta-analyses of randomised control trials and recommendations of clinical experts. *J Am Med Assoc* 1992;**268**:240–8.
2. Cochran WG, Cox GM. *Experimental designs*. Chichester: Wiley, 1992.
3. Cook TD, Campbell DT. *Quasi-experimentation: design and analysis issues for field settings*. Chicago: Rand McNally, 1979.
4. Anon. Search strategy. Effective professional practice module. In: *The Cochrane Database of Systematic Reviews*. Issue 3, 1997.
5. Whiting-O'Keefe QE, Henke C, Simborg DW. Choosing the correct unit of analysis in medical care experiments. *Med Care* 1984;**22**:1101–14.
6. Divine GW, Brown T, Frazier LM. The unit of analysis error in studies about physicians' patient care behaviour. *J Gen Intern Med* 1992;**7**:623–9.
7. Lomas J, Anderson GM, Domnick-Pierre K, Vayda E, Enkin MW, Hannah WJ. Do practice guidelines guide practice? *New Engl J Med* 1989;**321**:1306–11.
8. Evans CE, Haynes RB, Gilbert JR, Taylor DW, Sackett DL, Johnston M. Educational package on hypertension for primary care physicians. *Can Med Assoc J*. 1984;**130**:719–22.
9. Evans CE, Haynes RB, Birkett NJ *et al.* Does a mailed continuing program improve physician performance? Results of a randomised trial in anti-hypertensive care. *J Am Med Assoc* 1986;**255**:501–4.
10. Freemantle N, Harvey E, Grimshaw J, Wolf F, Oxman A, Grilli R, Bero L. The effectiveness of printed educational materials in changing the behaviour of healthcare professionals. In: Freemantle N, Bero L, Grilli R, Grimshaw J, Oxman A (eds), *Effective professional practice module. The Cochrane Database of Systematic Reviews*. Issue 3, 1996.
11. Covell DG, Uman GC, Manning PR. Information needs in office practice: are they being met? *Ann Intern Med* 1985;**103**:596–9.
12. Freemantle N, Wood J, Crawford F. Evidence into practice, experimentation and quasi experimentation: are the methods up to the task? *J Epidemiol Comm Health* 1998;**52**:75–81.
13. Rogers E. *Diffusion of innovations*. New York: Free Press, 1983.
14. Effective Health Care. Implementing clinical guidelines. Can guidelines be used to improve clinical practice? *Bulletin* No. 8. Leeds: University of Leeds, 1994.

15. North of England Study of Standards and Performance in General Practice. Medical audit in general practice: effects on doctors' clinical behaviour and the health of patients with common childhood conditions. *Br Med J* 1992;**304**: 1480.
16. Domenighetti G, Luraschi P, Casabianca A *et al*. Effect of information campaign by the mass media on hysterectomy rates. *Lancet* 1988;**ii**:1470–3.
17. Cornfield J. Randomisation by group: a formal analysis. *Am J Epidemiol* 1978; **108**:100–2.
18. Donner A, Birkett N, Buck C. Randomisation by cluster: sample size requirements and analysis. *Am J Epidemiol* 1981;**114**:906–14.
19. Donner A, Donald A. Analysis of data arising from a stratified design with the cluster as unit of randomisation. *Statist Med* 1987;**6**:43–52.
20. Donner A. A regression approach to the analysis of data arising from cluster randomisation. *Int J Epidemiol* 1985;**14**:322–6.
21. Donner A. Statistical methodology for paired cluster designs. *Am J Epidemiol* 1987;**126**:972–9.
22. LeLorier J, Grégoire G, Benhaddad A, Lapieere J, Derderian F. Discrepancies between meta analyses and subsequent large randomised, controlled trials. *New Engl J Med* 1997;**337**:536–42.
23. Smith TC, Spiegelhalter DJ, Thomas A. Bayesian approaches to random-effects meta analysis: a comparative study. *Statist Med* 1995;**14**:2685–99.
24. Hardy RJ, Thompson SG. A likelihood approach to meta analysis with random effects. *Statist Med* 1996;**15**:619–29.
25. Wolf FM. Meta-analysis: quantitative methods for research synthesis. In: *Quantitative applications in the social sciences*, No. 07–059. Newbury Park: Sage, 1986.
26. Hedges LV, Olkin I. *Statistical methods for meta analysis*. London: Academic Press, 1985.
27. Freemantle N, Haines A, Mason JM, Eccles M. CONSORT – an important step towards evidence based health care. *Ann Intern Med*, 1997;**126**:81–3.

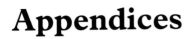

Appendices

I. What does "systematic" mean for reviews of methods?

JANE L HUTTON AND RICHARD ASHCROFT

Why is this an issue now?

Systematic reviews of scientific literature have always been important in scientific work, but only recently have they become a topic about which people have something to say. This is for two reasons. Firstly, a reasonable way to think about the systematic nature of a review is to suppose that "systematic" implies "completeness", but completeness is an unattainable ideal in most mature fields of research, given the huge and expanding range of journals, the variety of languages of publication, and the appreciable costs of reviewing. So methods of detecting and filtering literature have been invented and continue to be discussed and revised. Secondly, the reasons for doing systematic reviews have changed. Reviewing used to be done for two main reasons: graduate students obtaining and demonstrating a mastery of the field; and senior scientists summing up the state of the art in a field and stipulating or recommending the direction future research should follow. These reasons for review are still pertinent, but a third reason has come into prominence recently in health care: optimising practice (as distinct from research) in the light of the best evidence of effectiveness and efficiency.

Systematic reviews of methods have become an important issue as the quantity and forms of research done vary enormously and because optimal practice requires optimal reviewing. All areas of health care delivery and practice are now under scrutiny. Research methods are not, in principle, different from consideration of health care interventions. In both areas we can ask: Does this work? What constitutes best practice in systematic reviewing? Is the approach adopted by the Cochrane Collaboration a suitable model for systematic reviews of methods?

Defining "systematic review"

A systematic review is *systematic*: it involves rigorous application of a methodical search, compilation, and inference technique to the body of literature identified for review. This requires a system in the sense of a theory within which to organise data or knowledge. Equally obviously, a systematic review is a *review*. It is a survey of work done. As such, there are things that it cannot do. It will not do anything that requires new evidence, although it may answer, provisionally, new questions about old evidence. The questions it can answer are, however, largely determined by the questions which had been asked by the authors of the reviewed work. This can be frustrating, especially when a review is designed to answer some other question, not previously considered.

The purpose of a systematic review is to determine what is already known about some problem or technique. It should be thorough, identifying the relevant studies that meet specified standards of quality of evidence; and should be replicable, so that a review by another team, using the same standards and methods, should detect the same literature and come to the same factual conclusions. Of course, if the theoretical framework adopted by the reviewers is rejected, the conclusions might also be rejected.

Reviews of basic scientific research

The idea of a systematic review makes obvious good sense in scientific research. If one is working on subatomic physics, then to find out the current state of science, or interesting problems or controversies, one conducts a literature review. The first aim would be a big picture of the field, to see what was current. Then one would seek detail relevant to the topic selected from the big picture.

This is a research-driven model, a pragmatic approach to find an issue to work on, where "the answer" is not yet known. The first phase is usually pedagogical in function. The second phase might involve finding the current knowledge about an important physical constant, the methods used to measure it, and the values and margins of error attached to these methods. Typically one would have a theory of measurement and a theory of the relevant part of science in order to determine quality. This is a heuristic, and needs to be a good heuristic, given the time and money to be spent on research. The theory of the review would be guided by the currently accepted physical theory.

Reviews in health care

A systematic review in health care will share some features of a scientific review but differences will arise due both to the function of the review and the research methods used. Reviews might collect established facts not easily accessible, summarise knowledge and clinical norms on a topic, or help form judgements on whether clinical equipoise obtains on a given question.

Unlike reviews in physical science where the theory of the review is basically the relevant scientific theory, the theory of a review in health care is expressly methodological. Assessing the role of aspirin in reducing the risk of heart attack is usually done by considering statistical evidence from studies, rather than the biochemistry. To some extent the methods of randomised trials are such that reliability can be assessed without knowing much about the topic. Thus the theory of measurement dominates the review process.

Reviews of methods

During the preparation of the reviews in this book, it became clear that there were important differences between the different projects' source material and in the approaches used in detecting, compiling, and inferring from it. Some authors found huge quantities of material and their problem was to define criteria for cutting it down to manageable quantities. Other authors had very limited quantities of good quality material. For some, their project involved comparing the relevant merits of statistical techniques, while for others their problem was synthesising the results of psychological research. It became unclear whether the same techniques of systematic review would apply in all cases.

251

Content and purpose

Systematicity is therefore related to two main elements: content and purpose. The purpose of basic scientific and health care reviews differ, both in intent and in epistemology. In the scientific case, suppose we wish to measure G, the gravitational constant. The previous six or seven values differ. You do not do a meta-analysis of them but work out how to do a more accurate measurement, using the "old" values to calibrate the instruments used. In health care, the statistics on the accuracy of the measurement, or individual or collective uncertainty are important. An old value of G is just outdated and wrong.

In contrast, in statistics, earlier methods might not be wrong, just no longer relevant. Other methods remain relevant and a single reference to a good textbook is all that is needed in a review. Comprehensive lists of papers making small contributions to the theory presented in a textbook are irrelevant, whether one wishes to find out the current state of the subject, or to take theory further. An old randomised trial, if methodologically sound, remains a contribution to knowledge.

Determining the source material of the review

The domain about which information is required should be quite precisely defined. Any systematic review must begin by defining the body of literature which it is to review. This is not always easy. On the one hand, reviewing the evidence for the effectiveness of aspirin for secondary prevention of stroke may be fairly easy. On the other hand, the "basic science" approach had to be used by several of the reviews reported in this volume, in order to reach definitions of domain and content, as the initial search resulted in tens of thousands of references. For example, in the review of the implications of sociocultural contexts for the ethics of randomised trials (see Chapter 10), defining "relevance" proved difficult. Here, the technique used was to define three or four subquestions of clear salience to the main project proposal, which had well-defined literatures relating to them. These subquestions were then reviewed; systematically, the method of "explosion" was used (that is, generating an initial reference list, and then collecting the relevant works referenced by works on the initial list, and then works referenced by works on the new list, and so on) to construct a review of the main question, because the topic of the review had not been studied in its own right. By compiling results from related areas of research, a set of answers could be produced which could be relied on for defining areas where research was needed and for identifying areas in which sensitivity to ethical issues was needed. Findings derived in this way, however, are not as strong as might be derived from a new, empirical study dedicated to the question posed by the review. Equally, in the absence of such a study, the findings of the review are a reasonable basis for action because of the way the compilation and inference strategies were constructed.

Search methods

Searches often led to diminishing returns on information; an argument made well once is often enough, if not always to convince, at least to illustrate a point of view. The same argument rehearsed, with erratic quality, 100 times, is no more use the hundredth time than the first. Data gathered from 100 different situations, however, with at least an accepted minimum quality, weighs much more heavily than a single, localised, and isolated study.

Selection and compilation methods

A systematic review must have regard not only to the reliability of its methods of detecting relevant material, but also to the methods used in compiling what material it does gather and in drawing inferences from that compilation. There is now a large literature on meta-analysis of empirical studies which leads the way in the practice of systematic review. In a like manner, the Cochrane Collaboration's pragmatic rules for searching MEDLINE and other databases and for determining the relative quality of studies are now achieving widespread acceptance in reviews of randomised trials. The advantages of meta-analysis and of the Cochrane rules are clarity, applicability, acceptance (so that there is a common baseline standard) and, because the rules are algorithms for searching, any researcher can repeat them exactly, so that the material generated should be the same (up to the pre-set sampling reliability of the databases used).

Are these standards applicable outside reviews of empirical studies? In general, they are not. The first reason is simple enough: the Cochrane Collaboration rules are themselves methods which require assessment. There are fundamental disputes about the nature of science and the roles of knowledge, experience, and taste. Radical discoveries are often found by highly intelligent people using their instinct for harmony and beauty.

Methods work well because they are well adapted to the material. Vary the material and the adaptation varies too. Some reviews had to revise radically their criteria for assessing the quality of studies, as most articles failed to provide the information needed for the original assessment.

Conclusion

In general, the techniques of reviewing method differ from the techniques of reviewing empirical studies because what is being assessed is different. Rather than assessing the balance of evidence for the truth of some proposition, we are concerned with the reliability of a method or practical applicability or ethical legitimacy. In some cases, we may be concerned with mathematical proof. Some of these properties of a method may have measurable empirical content, so that a Cochrane Collaboration type of review is appropriate. We may be able to calibrate our methods against some agreed evidential standard and, where this can be done, it should be done. In general, the methods of detection and the completeness requirements of the search should be driven by the nature of the arguments that the review will make and by the uses the review will have.

II. Different types of systematic review in health services research

SARAH JL EDWARDS,
RICHARD J LILFORD AND SANDRA KIAUKA

The nature of reviews of methodological topics

Each review in this book is concerned with methods used to evaluate health technologies, rather than with the effectiveness of technologies. Such reviews of methodological topics are not the same as those concerned with clinical interventions, where numerical data on cure rates, diagnostic accuracy, or disease prevalence are aggregated across studies. In the case of methodological topics, there is no "gold standard" against which different methods may be compared. As a result, the choice between rival methods relies heavily on argument and ideas about, for example, how bias might be avoided, what is ethical, or what statistical methods are most appropriate. Therefore, a review of a methodological topic is likely to rely on extracting argument (perhaps as well as data) from the literature.

Many of the reviews contained sections in which topics of a numerical nature were reviewed, in which case, relatively standard methods could be used to summarise and assess the data. The fundamental difference between the reviews in this book and those dealing with health technologies is that the issues turn on ideas and theoretical discussion rather than on numbers and statistical analyses. In the case of the now familiar epidemiological reviews, such as those advocated by the Cochrane Collaboration, numerical data are brought together and assessed against methodological (quality) criteria. Similarly, arguments extracted from methodological papers must be categorised according to an intellectual framework and their validity assessed, at least in terms of starting premises. We will discuss the dangers inherent in this process, though it should be made clear that the nature of a review of a method is critically dependent on the topic in question. We will therefore begin by describing (and classifying) the types of review with which the authors in this book have had to grapple.

Types of review of methodological topics

The reviews in this book vary in terms of the questions posed and approach undertaken. The topics could be categorised by discipline (statistics, sociology, psychology, epidemiology, economics, ethics), but more basic distinctions relating to the type of literature analysed seemed to determine the nature of the review (or topic within a review). Some topics required analysis of quantitative data. Such data might be comparative (for example the effects of different methods of obtaining informed consent for randomised trials) or descriptive (for example attitudes of the public to randomised trials). Quantitative data were also sought in some reviews, not for their intrinsic value but for their methodological interest (for example, in Chapters 6 and 7 the results of randomised and non-randomised studies are compared within and between clinical topics). Yet other reviews rely on descriptive quantitative data (for example, case studies of how fast-changing technologies have come into widespread use). That said, articles were most often reviewed for ideas and theoretical and/or mathematical analyses, so that the literature was used as a data-source rather than a source of data.

Unsurprisingly, although interpretations of what a systematic review should look like varied by topic type, there was a common underlying idea that, in virtue of being systematic, a review should be "objective" and that the processes by which the literature were obtained and synthesised should be at once methodical and explicit. However, as previously mentioned, the kind of procedure used in the Cochrane Collaboration was simply not applicable to many topics. In such cases, the review methods necessarily had more in common with those of academic history or qualitative research generally than with those of quantitative scientists using a pre-determined algorithm to compare numerical findings and hence determine a "fact of the matter" about a technology's effectiveness.

Finding the material

All reviews took steps to uncover literature pertinent to a specific research question in a systematic and comprehensive way. In most cases, however, the initial algorithm was subject to a certain amount of trial and error. The predominant sources for most reviews were bibliographic databases. A review of a methodological topic may cover a number of different disciplines; for example, a review on the effects of participating in randomised trials might include both psychological and physical outcomes. As a result, reviewers searched a range of databases and, to use the above example, PsychINFO was relevant to psychological effects, while MEDLINE was a source of information on physical effects. Searching multiple databases overcame many limitations of single databases at the cost of considerable duplication of yield. Most of the well-established databases are based on a thesaurus and have associated problems with the accuracy of indexing. In addition, many methodological terms are not featured as keywords. There were further problems with text searches, mainly due to the existence of synonyms, homonyms, and acronyms to describe methodological concepts; for example, if you are interested in GCP (Good Clinical Practice) guidelines, you would retrieve articles on Granolocyte Chemotactic Protein, General Cystic Patterns, or even German Cardiovascular Prevention Study!

A prerequisite of any Cochrane Collaboration review is that research methods must be stated *a priori* and hence be independent of the data obtained, so that revisions to the protocol, once the review is under way, are strictly taboo. However, many of the reviews were forced to use an "iterative" approach, mainly because the literature was an unknown quantity at the time of the review's conception, but also because the topics rarely had well-defined boundaries. Searches on methodological topics frequently produced a vast yield of theoretical articles, where marginal returns of adding further articles decreased rapidly beyond a certain point. Sensible reviewers did not therefore pursue every last reference, but truncated their search when it appeared that new argument was no longer forthcoming – we refer to this as "theoretical saturation". It was therefore important to cast the net wide by searching many types of literature to make sure that a particular line of argument was not missed, rather than to pursue every instance of that argument. In this way, reviewers were able to make time for synthesis and writing up within the short duration of each project.

One of the valuable products of this programme is the vast record of literature, stored electronically, which is pertinent to a variety of methodological topics, and this can be tapped into and updated by future researchers. Indeed, some reviewers have already posted their databases on the World Wide Web for ease of access and in order to minimise duplication of effort where topics overlapped. It is important that future reviewers are aware of this resource.

Classification

In order to make sense of the information and argument in the reviewed literature, it was necessary to classify abstracted material. Authors therefore had to create an intellectual framework as the basis of the classification system. Since there are many different ways of classifying information, especially arguments dealing with ethical issues, a framework cannot be completely impartial. It is, however, explicit and hence open to scrutiny. In addition, all protocols were peer-reviewed to ensure that the suggested intellectual framework was sound.

Some projects employed more than one researcher to identify and classify information using predefined criteria so that interobserver reliability could be measured and different interpretations resolved. Interobserver reliability was more important for topics with ill-defined numerical outcomes (for example, what motivates people to participate in randomised trials) or where there was a risk that researchers would skew the review in a particular direction (for example, ethics of randomised trials). Some projects, such as is reported in Chapter 14 on Bayesian statistics, are arguably less vulnerable to such researcher biases and so were less concerned with formal measurement of interobserver reliability.

Analysis

The approach to analysis was dependent upon the type of review. A small number of reviews focused directly on comparative primary data and so resembled a Cochrane Collaboration type of review. For example, one of the reviews made a series of head-to-head comparisons of data obtained by randomised and by non-randomised studies. However, there was no example of a review where the subject matter was sufficiently homogeneous to be combined in a statistical meta-analysis. There were a number of reviews based on qualitative data – for example, a large number of studies in the ethics reviews described the attitudes of patients, the public and health care professionals to randomised trials in numerical terms. Again the studies were too heterogeneous to allow meaningful statistical combination of the data.

Most topics, however, consisted (entirely or mostly) of statistical techniques or philosophical arguments, highlighting points of agreement and controversy (perhaps offering explanations for the latter and using illustrative examples). As a result, the synthesis was qualitative. That is not to say that such synthesis lacked "objectivity". For example, in the review of ethics of randomised trials, two reviewers read the articles, independently classified the arguments, and produced a critique based on their internal consistency and the acceptability of their premises. Thus, interobserver reliability was estimated by independent reviewers producing syntheses (summaries) of the arguments, with authorial comment on the quality of those arguments where appropriate. Such "triangulation" of observers can reduce individual bias, but cannot offer protection against shared bias. To minimise the latter, the review also used a group of informed commentators against which to "test" their findings and arguments.

Index

pooling estimates 177–81
systematic reviews of 249–54
see also Bayesian methods;
consensus development
methods; implementation
methods; qualitative
methods; statistical methods
monitoring, Bayesian
methods 155–8
multi-attribute utility scales 24,
30–2
multiple testing 93–4
multistate survival analysis 165,
168–9

narrative review 243
needs-led methodological
research 3
NHS health technology
assessment programme 1–3
nominal group technique
(NGT) 201, 202, 203
non-health service costs 37
non-randomised trials
Bayesian methods 159
effect sizes 73–83
v. randomised trials 61–70
null hypothesis 100

objections, randomised
trials 110–11
off-the-shelf priors 155
one-way sensitivity analysis 188,
190
ordering, in questionnaires 52
organisation-based interventions,
evaluation 117–27
outcome measures, patient-
assessed 13–20
outcomes
appropriate 241
cluster-level
interventions 117–18, 119
intermediate 87–9

measurement of 5–6
randomised trials 103
outliers, consensus development
methods 208, 209
overinterpretation, consent
failure 113

parallel group designs 89
participant observation 130, 239
participants
consensus-based
guidelines 205–6
recruitment 91
participation
differences in 66–7
invitations 100–2
patient and clinician 90, 91
partitioned survival analysis 166–7
paternalism 112, 113–14
patient data, re-analysing 181–3
patient outcome measures,
implementation trials 241
patient participation 90, 91
patient preference 67–8, 82
patient questionnaires 46–57
patient-assessed outcome
measures 13–20
patient-level cost data 193–4
patients, effects of randomised
trials 102–3
performance bias 89
pharmaceutical industry,
guidelines 144
physical functioning
dimension 24, 29
placebo-controlled randomised
trials 100
placebos 92
population, evaluative
studies 62–3, 69
posterior distribution 152, 153,
154–5
poverty, randomised trials 110,
114